Techniques of measurement in medicine: 4
Series Editor: Dr B. Watson
Department of Medical Electronics
St Bartholomew's Hospital, London
Consultant Editor: Professor J. Rotblat

An introduction to radiation dosimetry

An introduction to radiation dosimetry

S. LOVELL

Medical College of St Bartholomew's Hospital, London

Cambridge University Press

CAMBRIDGE

LONDON · NEW YORK · MELBOURNE

CAMBRIDGE UNIVERSITY PRESS
Cambridge, New York, Melbourne, Madrid, Cape Town,
Singapore, São Paulo, Delhi, Tokyo, Mexico City

Cambridge University Press
The Edinburgh Building, Cambridge CB2 8RU, UK

Published in the United States of America by Cambridge University Press, New York

www.cambridge.org
Information on this title: www.cambridge.org/9780521294973

First published 1979
Re-issued 2011

A catalogue record for this publication is available from the British Library

Library of Congress Cataloguing in Publication data

Lovell, S.
An introduction to radiation dosimetry.

(Techniques of measurement in medicine; 4)
Bibliography: p.
Includes index.
1. Radiation dosimetry. 1. Title. 11. Series.
QC795.32.R3L68   539.7′7   78-67261

ISBN 978-0-521-22436-9 Hardback
ISBN 978-0-521-29497-3 Paperback

Contents

To Andrew Timothy and Simon Piers
hoping that they too may derive satisfaction
from the physical world

Preface

In this book I have attempted to develop an elementary introduction to radiation dosimetry. I have used only the modern units
of dosimetry but have referred to older, obsolescent units and,
where necessary, given conversion factors. In defining the units I
have used the δ notation throughout to represent a small quantity
of energy, mass or charge, instead of the differential notation used
by the International Commission on Radiation Units. I feel that
this notation is in more common use in scientific work and is
easier for a beginner to understand.

A host of different effects of radiation have been used at
various times as the basis of dosemeters but I have confined
myself to only those which are at present used extensively, and
even with these effects I have tended to keep to the principles and
have avoided minutiae.

With such a physical subject a certain amount of mathematics
has crept in since physicists use mathematics as part of their
language. I have kept the mathematics as simple as possible and
have used it only where I feel its use is essential to explain a point
without having to resort to the use of a great many words. Those
readers who are not at ease with this particular language need not
follow the derivations in detail but may leap-frog to the results
that they lead to. Those who understand the language should gain
a greater insight into the subject by following the individual steps.

London, 1978

1. Some introductory ideas

The structure of the atom

A neutral atom comprises a small, positively charged nucleus surrounded by shells of electrons. The nucleus consists of protons
and neutrons. The masses of the proton and neutron are approximately equal, the neutron having a slightly greater mass than the
proton. Since the charge on an electron is equal in magnitude but
opposite in sign to that on a proton, the total number of electrons
in the shells of a neutral atom is equal to the number of protons
in its nucleus. This number is equal to the atomic number (Z) of
the atom. The mass of an electron is of the order of one two-
thousandth of that of a proton and consequently most of the
mass of an atom is due to its nucleus. Whereas atoms have radii
about 10^{-10} metres, nuclear radii are about 10^{-15} metres.

The arrangement of electrons in shells in an atom is shown in
fig. 1. The K shell contains two electrons, the L shell eight, the M
shell eighteen, and so on. The atom with the lowest atomic number, hydrogen, has a single electron in its K shell. Next above
hydrogen is helium, with two electrons in its K shell. Lithium,
with atomic number 3, has two electrons in its K shell and one in
its L shell, and so on.

Shells from the L shell outwards are subdivided into subshells.
The nomenclature of the shells (K, L, M, etc.) may seem rather
whimsical; it originates from the notation of the early workers in
spectroscopy who used this system to classify the spectra produced
by atoms, before the significance of quantum numbers was under-
stood.

The quantum theory of radiation

We will be dealing throughout this book with electromagnetic

Fig. 1

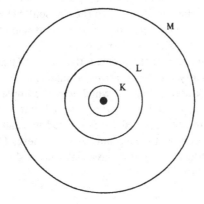

radiation, examples of which, in order of decreasing wavelength, are radio waves, infrared radiation, visible light, ultraviolet light, X-rays and γ-rays. They are essentially the same type of radiation, being an electric and a magnetic field both of which oscillate with time. The vectors which represent the electric and magnetic fields are perpendicular to each other and to the direction of propagation of the wave. These radiations can all be transmitted from one point to another without a tangible connection between the two points. In a vacuum they all travel with the same velocity (approximately 3×10^8 metres per second). The relationship between the wavelength (λ), the frequency of oscillation (ν) and the velocity of propagation c is

$$\nu\lambda = c$$

The apparent differences in character, differences in interaction with matter and mode of detection, of waves from the various parts of the electromagnetic spectrum arise from their different frequencies. Visible light, for instance, readily stimulates the eye, whereas the long wavelength radio waves used in radio transmission do not.

All wave disturbances show certain characteristic properties. In particular, they can be diffracted by objects or apertures whose dimensions are comparable with their wavelength.

Up to the end of the nineteenth century most of the known properties of electromagnetic waves were explained by Maxwell's electromagnetic theory. One of the principal features of this theory is that radiation is produced continuously by a source. If, say, an aerial is connected to a radio transmitter and the flow of energy is measured at some point, it will be found that the energy flow is continuous. There will be periodic fluctuations in the response of the detector due to the sinusoidal character of the waves, but, nevertheless, these fluctuations will follow continuously and regularly one after another.

About the end of the nineteenth century, Planck, while working on a theory for the spectrum of radiation emitted by a black body, introduced a concept which was at complete variance with the electromagnetic theory. He proposed that, instead of radiation being emitted continuously, it is emitted in small discrete packets or quanta. The relationship between the energy (E) of a quantum and the frequency (ν) of the associated wave disturbance is given by the relationship

$$E = h\nu$$

where h is a universal constant, called Planck's constant, of value 6.63×10^{-34} joule second. Embodied in this equation is an apparent contradiction. The radiation has some of the properties of a wave (frequency) and yet behaves as a particle (has a discrete energy). This dual nature of radiation is ever present and which of the two characteristics predominates depends on the frequency or quantum energy. Long wavelength radiations, such as radio waves, tend to behave almost exclusively as waves. As one goes to higher frequencies the quantum nature becomes more pronounced. Visible light behaves as a wave in most of its interactions, but in the ejection of photoelectrons from a metal surface it behaves as a stream of particles. Radiations of higher frequency than visible light tend to behave more predominantly as particles. X-rays, for example, interact with matter almost exclusively as particles (and yet they can be diffracted by a crystal lattice). Visible light is roughly the boundary between the quantum and wave nature of electromagnetic radiation, radiations of lower frequency tending to behave predominantly as waves and radiations of higher frequency tending to exhibit a particulate nature. To be in keeping with the terminology of the other particles of atomic and nuclear physics a special name has been coined for the quanta of radiation: they are called photons. In contrast with most of the other fundamental particles, the photon has zero mass.

One may expect that, since radiations, which are normally thought of as being waves, act in some circumstances as particles, the converse would be true and entities which are normally considered to be particles may behave as waves. This has been demonstrated experimentally with a number of atomic particles. For instance, electrons, which show typical properties of a particle (such as mass), can be diffracted by a crystal lattice in much the same way as light is diffracted by a diffraction grating.

The energy levels of isolated atoms

A great deal of experimental data, derived principally from spectroscopy, indicates that a stationary, isolated atom cannot have a continuously variable energy. Its energy is quantized and the atom can only have certain discrete energy levels. These levels are shown schematically in fig. 2. The diagram is really a graph with only one axis, energy, plotted vertically. Each line represents an allowed energy level of the atom, the spaces between the lines being forbidden energy values.

The sketch is drawn for hydrogen, the simplest atom, with a single electron. The levels and the spacings between them are different for atoms of the different chemical elements but are identical for all atoms of a particular isotope. The lowest of the levels (E_1) is the least energy that the stationary atom can have and is called the ground state. If the atom is subjected to a suitable stimulus, for example by irradiating it with a beam of charged particles of variable energy, it will be found that, as the energy of the particles is increased, a stage is reached when the atom jumps from the ground state to the energy level E_2. This occurs when the energy of the particles is just equal to $E_2 - E_1$. During this transition the electron jumps from its normal orbit to one farther from the nucleus. If the energy of the bombarding particles is less than $E_2 - E_1$ the atom will remain in its ground state and receive no energy from the particles, no matter how intense the beam of particles is made.

If the energy of the particles is further increased, a stage is reached when another transition can occur. In this case the atom jumps from the ground state to the level E_3, when the energy of the particles is equal to $E_3 - E_1$, and the electron moves into an orbit still more remote from the nucleus. As the energy of the particles is further increased, the atom can be excited into each of the series of energy levels of fig. 2.

Only the first few energy levels of the atom are indicated in fig. 2, the upper levels getting closer and closer together. In each successive level the electron is moved farther and farther from the nucleus but still remains attached to it. This situation cannot continue indefinitely since, if the atom is given sufficient energy, the electron will become detached from the nucleus (or is removed infinitely far from the nucleus); this is the significance of E_∞. The

Fig. 2

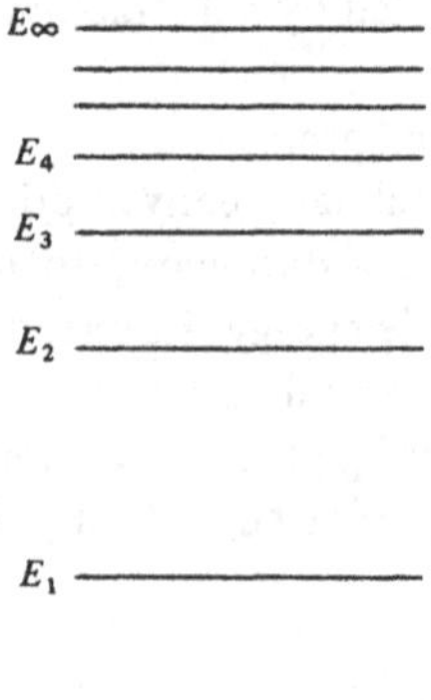

E_∞ ————————

E_4 ————————

E_3 ————————

E_2 ————————

E_1 ————————

energy difference $E_\infty - E_1$ is the amount of energy that has to be supplied to the atom in order just to remove the electron from the attraction of the nucleus. Any energy supplied above this level is acquired by the electron in the form of kinetic energy. If the electron is removed from the sphere of influence of the nucleus the atom is said to be ionized. The least amount of energy required to ionize the atom is $E_\infty - E_1$. In the case of the hydrogen atom, this is about 2.18×10^{-18} joules.

If the atom has been excited into an energy level above the ground state, it is in an unstable condition. Any physical system tends to adopt a configuration with least energy in order to become stable. As an example, if the bob of a pendulum is pulled aside its energy is increased by doing work against the gravitational field. When the bob is released it is unstable and in order to minimize its gravitational energy and become stable it swings back to its resting position. The same effect occurs with an excited atom; it returns to the ground state. In so doing it has to rid itself of its surplus energy. This it does by radiating a photon of energy equal to the difference in energy between the excited state and the ground state. If the atom has been excited to the energy level E_3, the energy of the photon is given by

$$hv = E_3 - E_1$$

where once again h is Planck's constant and v is the frequency of the waves associated with the photon. Since the energy levels of the atoms of a particular chemical element are specific to that element, so also will be the frequencies and wavelengths of the photons emitted when its atoms are excited by a suitable stimulus. This is the origin of the characteristic optical and X-ray spectra of atoms.

The minimum amount of energy required to remove a particular electron from an atom is called its binding energy. In a high atomic number atom the K electrons are tightly bound to the nucleus owing to the high nuclear charge and the small distance separating the electrons from the nucleus. The electrons in the various L subshells are less tightly bound because they are farther away from the nucleus. The M electrons are still less tightly bound. The outermost, valence electrons are the least tightly bound of all. Ionization of an atom occurs most easily by removal of the valence electrons. Much higher amounts of energy have to be supplied to remove the innermost electrons. The binding energy of electrons in a particular shell increases with the atomic number of the atom owing to the increased attraction of its nuclear charge.

Units of energy used in atomic and nuclear physics

Although the international unit of energy is the joule (J), a more convenient unit, the electron volt (eV), is used in atomic and nuclear physics. The electron volt is the amount of energy that a particle with the same charge as an electron, 1.6×10^{-19} coulombs (C), gains as it passes through a potential difference of 1 volt (V). The practical advantage of this unit is that it allows one readily to specify the energy of a particle that has been accelerated by allowing it to pass between two electrodes at different potentials in a vacuum. If, say, an electron were accelerated between electrodes at a potential difference of 300 V, the energy gained by the electron would be 300 eV. Furthermore, since the charge on all atomic particles is a simple multiple of the charge on the electron, the unit is easily applied to any charged particle. For instance if a helium nucleus (with charge twice that on the electron) were accelerated through a 300 V potential difference its energy would be 600 eV. The use of the unit has been extended to specify the energy of uncharged particles such as neutrons and photons. It has a number of multiples, the more important of which are the kilo-electron volt (keV) and million electron volt (MeV); thus 1 keV equals 10^3 eV and 1 MeV equals 10^6 eV. The conversion factor from electron volts to joules can be derived from the relationship for the amount of work done when a charge Q coulombs passes through a potential difference of V volts,

$$\text{Work} = QV \text{ J}$$

Since the charge on an electron is 1.6×10^{-19} C,

$$1 \text{ eV} = 1.6 \times 10^{-19} \times 1 = 1.6 \times 10^{-19} \text{ J}$$

and similarly,

$$1 \text{ MeV} = 1.6 \times 10^{-13} \text{ J}$$

Predictions of the special theory of relativity

Although we need not be deeply involved in the underlying philosophy of the theory of relativity, some of its predictions are relevant in the field of radiation dosimetry. There is ample experimental evidence in the field of atomic and nuclear physics for the validity of these predictions. In Newtonian mechanics the mass of a particle is considered to be a constant, invariable quantity. In relativistic mechanics the mass of a particle depends on its velocity in the following way:

$$m = m_0 \left[1 - \left(\frac{v}{c}\right)^2\right]^{-\frac{1}{2}}$$

where m is the mass of the particle when its velocity is v, m_0 is its mass when it is at rest and c is the velocity of light. The form of this variation of m with v is shown in fig. 3. For values of v small compared with the velocity of light, m is constant and equal to m_0. As v increases the value of m also increases, tending to infinity as v approaches c. The velocities we meet in everyday life are usually small compared with the velocity of light and the mass of a particle is constant with a value m_0, as is assumed in Newtonian mechanics. In atomic and nuclear physics the particles dealt with have small rest masses and can easily be accelerated to velocities which are an appreciable fraction of the velocity of light. In these circumstances their mass is no longer constant. As an example, an electron (of rest mass 9.1×10^{-31} kg) accelerated between electrodes at a potential difference of 30 kV has a velocity of the order of thirty per cent of the velocity of light and its mass is about six per cent greater than its rest mass. If the accelerating voltage is increased to 200 kV, typical of the accelerating voltages in X-ray tubes used in radiotherapy, the velocity of the electron is about fifty per cent of the velocity of light and its mass about twenty per cent greater than its rest mass. If the electron is accelerated to an energy of 15 MeV, equivalent to accelerating it with a potential difference of fifteen million volts, its velocity is 0.9995 of the velocity of light and its mass is of the order of thirty times its rest mass.

Fig. 3
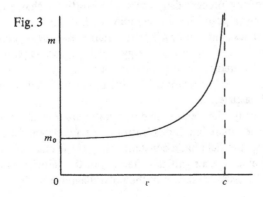

Another prediction of the theory of relativity is that mass and energy can be converted into each other. The relationship between energy (E) in joules and mass (m) in kilograms is

$$E = m\,c^2$$

where c is the velocity of light in metres per second. What this equation means is that if a mass m of matter were completely converted into energy, the amount of energy produced would be equal to $m\,c^2$. For instance, when a kilogram of matter is converted to energy the amount of energy produced is equal to 9×10^{16} J. One can look upon mass as a highly concentrated form of energy and, in the previous example of relativistic effects, where the mass of a particle increases with its velocity, one can look upon the increase in energy as the cause of the increase in mass.

In chemical reactions it is found, by direct weighing, that the total mass of the reacting species is the same before and after the reaction, although energy may be released or absorbed during the process. This apparent contradiction of the theory of relativity arises from the small energy change and the crudeness of the weighing system. The change of energy involved in chemical reactions is negligible compared with the total energy-equivalent of the masses of the reactants and consequently the change of mass is too small to be detected with a chemical balance. If a process is chosen where the energy change is significant compared with the masses involved, the mass change can be easily detected. An example of such a reaction is the process of pair production (p. 33) which occurs when high energy photons are absorbed in matter. In this process, when a photon enters the field near the nucleus of an atom, the photon (energy) may disappear and in its place a pair of oppositely charged particles (mass) is created. The inverse of this process also occurs. The positively charged member of the pair (a positron) may combine with an electron and the two particles annihilate each other, their masses being converted to an equivalent amount of energy which appears as photons.

The last prediction of the theory of relativity which impinges on dosimetry is the relativistic distortion of the electric field of a charged particle.

Classically, the electric field of a static point charge is given by the inverse square law and is isotropic. At a constant distance from the charge the field has a constant value. If the charge is in motion, and its velocity is a significant fraction of the velocity of light, the field is distorted, as shown in the polar diagrams of fig. 4. In these diagrams the electric intensity at an angle θ to the direction of motion of the charge is proportional to the length of a vector drawn from the origin, O, at an angle θ to the path of the charge, until it meets the curve under consideration. The various distributions are symmetrical about the path of the particle; the three-dimensional distribution may be obtained by rotating the diagram about the direction of motion of the charge. It will be seen that in the classical case ($v/c \sim 0$) the distribution is isotropic. As the velocity of the charge increases, the electric intensity decreases in the forward and backward direction ($\theta = 0$ and $\theta = 180°$) and increases in a direction at right angles to the path of the charge. This distortion of the field increases with increasing velocity of the charge. It will also be noticed that the distributions are symmetrical about $\theta = 90°$; the reduction of the field in front of the charge ($\theta = 0$) and behind it ($\theta = 180°$) is equal and one cannot tell from the shape of the distributions whether the charge is moving from left to right or in the opposite direction.

The importance of this relativistic field distortion in dosimetry lies in the fact that at high velocities the distance at which the field of a charged particle can interact with atoms of an absorber, and be effective in transferring energy to them, is greater than when the velocity is low. As the particle passes through the absorber it sweeps out a cylindrical volume throughout which its field is capable of transferring energy to the atoms. The radius of this cylinder is greater at high velocities and consequently more atoms are affected by the particle.

Fig. 4

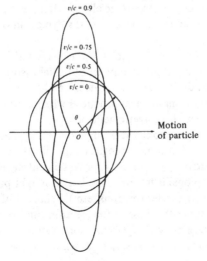

2. Ionizing radiations and their inter-action with matter at the atomic level

Ionizing radiations are radiations which are capable of ionizing neutral matter as they pass through it. They include X-rays and γ-rays and particles such as alpha particles, beta particles and neutrons. The current trend is to refer to them all as particles since X-rays and γ-rays interact with matter as though they were particulate, especially in the interactions which lead to ionization.

Ionizing radiations are subdivided into directly ionizing radiations, such as alpha particles and beta particles, and indirectly ionizing radiations, such as X-rays and neutrons. Particles of this latter group produce most of their ionization by first producing a charged particle which then ionizes matter as it passes through it. The term indirectly ionizing radiation is a slight overstatement of the case, since these radiations, by the very fact that they produce a charged particle in neutral matter, must ionize directly to some extent.

In considering the interaction of ionizing radiations with matter they are best divided into four groups: heavy charged particles (such as alpha particles), light charged particles (such as electrons), photons and neutrons.

The interaction of heavy charged particles with matter
Heavy charged particles include protons, deuterons, alpha particles and other atomic nuclei, and, in the context of their ionization of matter, mesons.

Alpha particles are the nuclei of helium atoms. They are produced during the radioactive disintegration of some nuclei or they may be produced by artificially accelerating helium nuclei to high energies in an accelerator such as a cyclotron or a Van de Graaff accelerator.

Deuterons are the nuclei of the heavy stable isotope of hydrogen and protons are the nuclei of its light isotope. They are not produced during radioactive decay and must be accelerated artificially. Protons are also produced when hydrogenous material is irradiated with energetic neutrons.

Mesons are produced in some nuclear reactions. The π meson is of interest in some biological experiments; it may have either unit positive or negative charge or be neutral. The mass of π mesons (pions) is intermediate between light particles (electrons) and heavy particles (protons, etc.), being about two hundred and seventy times the mass of the electron. Biological interest centres on the negatively charged π meson. As a negative pion passes through matter and is slowed down it may be captured by an

oppositely charged atomic nucleus, leading to a catastrophic disintegration of the nucleus into a number of charged fragments
which produce a high deposition of energy locally.

The energy spectrum of alpha particles from a radioactive
source is a line spectrum (fig. 5). It may consist of a single line or
more, depending on the decay scheme of the parent nucleus. The
energies of alpha particles from radioactive sources are rarely less
than 4 MeV or greater than 9 MeV.

Particles which have been accelerated artificially have an energy
spectrum similar to that of fig. 6, the energy spread and the shape
of the curve depending on the characteristics of the accelerator.

When heavy charged particles pass through matter two processes, apart from nuclear interactions, can occur. These processes
are radiative and inelastic collisions. In a radiative collision the
particle is accelerated in the electric field near the nucleus and
loses energy by radiating a photon. Since the masses of the heavy

Fig. 5

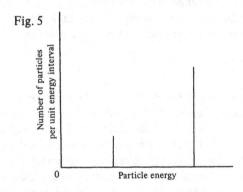

Fig. 6

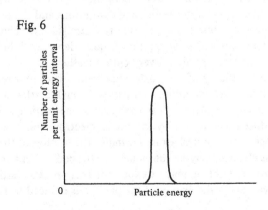

charged particles are large, the acceleration is small and radiative energy loss can usually be neglected except at very high energies.

In an inelastic collision the field of the particle interacts with the electrons of the atoms of the absorbing matter and transfers energy to them. If the energy transfer is small the atom is raised to an excited state. With larger energy transfer the electron may be detached completely from the atom causing ionization. If the energy transfer is sufficiently in excess of the binding energy of the electron in the atom, the excess energy is given to the electron as kinetic energy and the electron may be able to produce further excitation and ionization on its own account, in which case it is termed a delta ray or secondary electron. Delta rays are always produced with a component of velocity in the same direction as the incident particle. The highest energy delta rays travel in the same direction as the incident particle. Delta rays with lower energy diverge at an angle from the path of the particle, the greater the angle the lower the energy of the delta ray.

The maximum amount of energy that a heavy charged particle can lose in a single inelastic collision is of the order of

$$4\left(\frac{m}{M}\right)E$$

where m is the mass of the electron and M is the mass of the incident particle of energy E. For protons this is of the order of $E/500$ and for alpha particles about $E/2000$. During collisions having these maximum energy transfers, in which a delta ray is produced, the incident particle is deflected only very slightly from its course. Most of the collisions are of much lower energy transfer and the deflection of the particle is correspondingly even less. For this reason the energy loss of the particle as it passes through matter is fairly smooth and continuous and the path of the particle is a close approximation to a straight line. The ionization produced by the particle is quite dense, with individual pairs of ions being produced very close together.

When the energy of the particle has been sufficiently reduced, by ionization and excitation as it passes through matter, a further effect takes place. Although the velocity of the particle has not been reduced to zero, it may capture an electron from the absorber and proceed as a neutral atom. Owing to the motion of the particle this electron may be subsequently stripped off and at a later stage another electron may be captured. This process continues until, eventually, the energy of the particle is reduced to the thermal energy of the surrounding matter. In the case of the alpha particle two electrons may be captured and lost. The greater the charge of the particle, the higher is the energy at which capture and loss occurs. Theoretical treatment of the region of capture and loss is difficult. It will be noted that in this region the effective charge of the particle is reduced by the presence of the captured electron and so its interaction with the absorber is lessened.

The theoretical treatment of energy loss of the particle above the region of capture and loss of electrons is sound and shows good agreement with experimental measurement. The relationships derived by Bethe for the rate of change of the energy (E) of the particle with respect to distance (x) along its path are

$$-\frac{\mathrm{d}E}{\mathrm{d}x} = \frac{4\pi e^4 z^2}{mv^2}NB \tag{1}$$

with

$$B = Z\ln(2mv^2/I) \tag{1a}$$

for non-relativistic velocities and

$$B = Z\left[\ln(2mv^2/I) - \ln(1-\beta^2) - \beta^2\right] \tag{1b}$$

for relativistic velocities.

In these relationships v is the velocity and ze the charge of the incident particle, e and m are respectively the charge and mass of the electron, N is the number of atoms per unit volume of the absorber, Z is the atomic number of the absorber and I is the mean excitation energy of its atoms. β is the ratio v/c where c is the velocity of light.

$\mathrm{d}E/\mathrm{d}x$ is called the stopping power of the medium. It will be seen that the relativistic expression tends to the non-relativistic relation for small values of β. The general shape of this expression is shown in fig. 7. The sharp drop with increasing energy in the low energy region comes from the $1/v^2$ term in equation 1; the flat minimum originates from the $1/v^2$ term not varying very much as v tends towards c. The relativistic rise originates partly from the fact that the maximum energy the particle can transfer at a single inelastic collision increases with its energy and partly from the relativistic distortion of its electric field extending its range of effectiveness, thus encompassing a larger number of atoms.

The main use of these expressions is as interpolation formulae in deriving range—energy relationships from experimental measurements at discrete energies. The equations can be integrated to give the distance the particle travels in the absorber as its energy changes from E_1 to E_2.

The theoretical treatment used in deriving equations 1, 1a and 1b is slightly in error. The method of calculation treats the interaction of the charged particle with an isolated atom of the absorber and then the total effect of the absorber is found by multiplying this result by the number of atoms per unit volume. This treatment neglects the fact that condensing the isolated atoms together may influence the effect of the field of the particle on more distant atoms. In fig. 8, which represents a condensed medium, as the particle passes atom B its charge tends to polarize this atom and the polarized atom B then reduces the field of the particle at atom A, causing a reduction of the interaction of the particle on A. The effect is known as the density effect since it depends on the number of atoms per unit volume of the medium. The density effect becomes more important at high velocities where the relativistic distortion of the field of the particle makes it effective over a greater range. The density effect is least in gases, where the atoms are far apart. To allow for the density effect a small term δ

Fig. 7

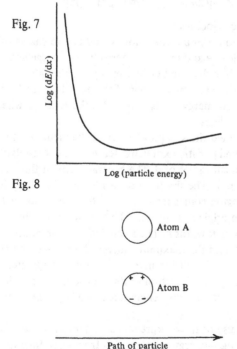

Log (particle energy)

Fig. 8

should be subtracted inside the square brackets of equation 1*b*.
δ is usually quite small for heavy charged particles but may be
appreciable for electrons of comparable energy since their
velocities are much higher.

Measurements of the absorption of a beam of heavy charged
particles may be made using the experimental arrangement shown
in fig. 9, employing a detector which responds to the number of
particles incident upon it and recording the variation of detector
response as the thickness of the absorber is increased. The variation
is illustrated in fig. 10. The wide range of thickness over which
the detector response is constant is due to the very low scattering
of the particles as they pass through matter. An initially parallel
beam of these particles stays substantially parallel as it is absorbed,
and few particles are scattered out of the beam. The sudden drop
in detector response occurs as the particles are brought to rest.
The range of a particle is the total thickness of absorber it traverses before it is brought to rest. The ranges of all the particles in
a monoenergetic beam are not identical. Since the energy transfer
at each collision of an individual particle is discrete and varies
from near zero up to the maximum allowed for the particle, the
individual ranges show a small spread about a mean value, as indicated in fig. 10. If the energy transfer at each collision were very
small and the particles were not deflected at all at each collision,

Fig. 9

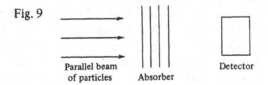

Parallel beam   Absorber   Detector
of particles

Fig. 10

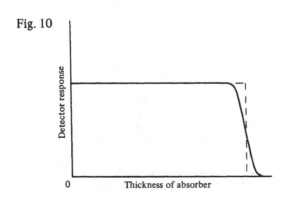

the response would follow the broken line and all the particles would have identical ranges.

The range of particles in a particular medium increases with their energy and decreases with the charge on the particle. Alpha particles with two units of charge have a smaller range than protons of the same energy. To give an idea of orders of magnitude, alpha particles from radioactive sources are stopped by a few sheets of paper or a few centimetres of air.

If the specific ionization (amount of ionization per unit distance) along the path of a beam of heavy charged particles is measured, the distribution is given by the Bragg curve shown in fig. 11. The rise towards the end of the path of the particles is due to the reduction in the energy of the particles and, as is shown in fig. 7, the accompanying increase in the rate of energy loss. The cause of the shape of the curve after the peak is twofold; it is partly due to the spread of ranges of the individual particles and partly due to the electron capture and loss phenomenon reducing the effective charge of the particles. The peak in the Bragg curve for negative pions is enhanced by the ionization of the particles emitted during nuclear disintegration following capture of the pion.

The interaction of light charged particles with matter
The group of light charged particles consists of electrons and positrons. They may be produced during radioactive disintegration or when photons interact with matter (pp. 25–39). High energy electrons with a small energy spread may be produced by accelerating electrons from a heated filament in an accelerator such as a betatron, a linear accelerator, or a synchrotron. A typical energy spectrum of beta particles from a radioactive source is shown in

Fig. 11

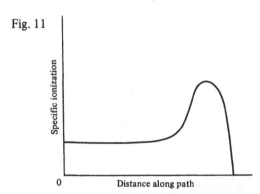

fig. 12. In contrast with the characteristic line spectrum of alpha particles there is a continuous variation of energy from zero up to a maximum energy E_{max}. This continuous spectrum is due to the simultaneous emission of an antineutrino during the nuclear disintegration. Values of E_{max} of the known β^- emitters range from less than 10 keV to more than 13 MeV. The spectrum of electrons from an accelerator is similar to that shown for heavy particles in fig. 6.

When electrons pass through matter they are subject to both inelastic and radiative collisions. The role of radiative collisions is more important for electrons than heavy charged particles since their acceleration is very much greater in the field around the nucleus. Indeed, energy loss due to radiation, or bremsstrahlung as it is called, is the dominant factor in the energy loss of fast electrons, particularly in high atomic number absorbers.

The theoretical treatment of energy loss due to inelastic collisions is similar to that of heavy particles except that in this case the density correction is larger and allowance must be made for the masses of the two interacting particles being the same. The expressions derived for the stopping power are similar to, but rather more complicated than, those given for heavy particles on p. 13. The masses of the two particles being equal leads to the important consequence that the incident particle may suffer large energy losses during individual collisions and be deflected through large angles. Since the two particles emerging from a collision of high energy transfer are both electrons, the particle with the higher energy is taken as the primary particle and hence the maximum energy transfer in a collision is half the kinetic energy of the incident particle. Owing to the large energy transfers and correspondingly large deflections of the particle, the path of an electron in

Fig. 12

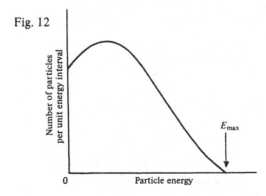

matter is tortuous and the path length does not approximate to
the range measured experimentally as the thickness of material
which will bring the particle to rest. Experimental measurements
of the range of electrons of different energies give poor agreement
with theory. The situation is made worse by multiple elastic
scattering of the electron by atoms of the absorber, where the
electron is deflected by an atom without loss of energy.

During a radiative collision the electron enters the Coulomb
field near the nucleus and is accelerated by the force exerted upon
it. One of the predictions of the electromagnetic theory is that an
accelerated charge emits radiation. The emission by an electron in
the field of the nucleus is a quantum effect; the energy is radiated
as a single photon and the electron suffers a step-like change of
energy. The process is illustrated in fig. 13. If the kinetic energy
of the electron is E_1 before and E_2 after the collision, the energy
of the photon is given by the relationship

$$h\nu = E_1 - E_2$$

E_2 can take any value between zero and E_1; thus a continuous
spectrum of photon energies is produced when a beam of electrons
strikes matter (fig. 14). The upper energy limit of this spectrum
occurs when $E_2 = 0$, when the whole of the kinetic energy of the

Fig. 13

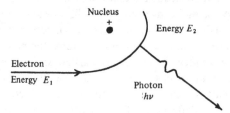

Fig. 14

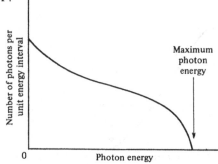

electron is converted to a photon. The energy of the photons produced lies in the X-ray region of the electromagnetic spectrum.
This is the principal mechanism of production of X-rays in X-ray
sets, where a beam of electrons is accelerated and allowed to
strike a target.

The angular distribution of the radiation is illustrated in the
polar diagrams of fig. 15. The three-dimensional distribution of
the radiation is obtained by rotating the diagram about the path
of the electron. With low energy electrons the radiation is produced predominantly at right angles to the path of the electron.
At higher energies the lobes swing forward until they eventually
coalesce at high energies into a single lobe with the maximum
intensity in the same direction as the electron was moving. Both
figs. 14 and 15 are drawn for very thin targets. In a thick target
the distributions are modified by the scattering of the electrons,
their loss of energy due to inelastic collisions, the probability of
suffering more than one radiative collision and the attenuation of
the radiation in the material of the target.

A further mechanism by which electrons can produce X-rays is
illustrated in fig. 16. The incident electron transfers sufficient
energy to one of the electrons bound in an inner shell of the atom
and ejects it completely from the atom leaving a hole in the inner
shell. The hole is then filled by an electron dropping in from one
of the outer shells. Since the outer electrons are less tightly bound
than the inner electrons, the electron dropping in to the hole has
a surplus of energy and radiates a photon during the transition.
Once again, the photon energy lies in the X-ray region of the
electromagnetic spectrum. Since the binding energies of the electrons in an atom depend on its atomic number, the radiation produced is characteristic of the atoms of the absorbing material.

Fig. 15

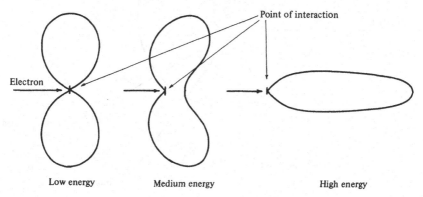

Low energy   Medium energy   High energy

Characteristic radiation is used in X-ray crystallography to investigate the structure of matter. The characteristic spectrum is superimposed on the continuous spectrum shown in fig. 14 as a series of lines. The energy loss of electrons by this process is usually negligible compared with loss by inelastic collisions and bremsstrahlung.

Measurements of the absorption of electrons using the experimental arrangement of fig. 9 are difficult to interpret because various end-points are used to specify the range of particles. If beta particles from a radioactive source are used the curve shown in fig. 17 is obtained. In this diagram the logarithm of the detector response is plotted against the thickness of the absorber. The first part of the curve approximates to an exponential absorption. The long tail is caused by bremsstrahlung produced in the absorber.

When monoenergetic electrons are used the absorption curves of fig. 18 are produced. These curves show a substantially straight portion followed by a tail. The straight portion can be extrapolated to yield an extrapolated range.

The Bragg curve produced when the ionization in matter along the axis of a beam of initially parallel, monoenergetic electrons is measured does not show the marked peak that is obtained with heavy particles. The reason for this difference is that the electrons

Fig. 16

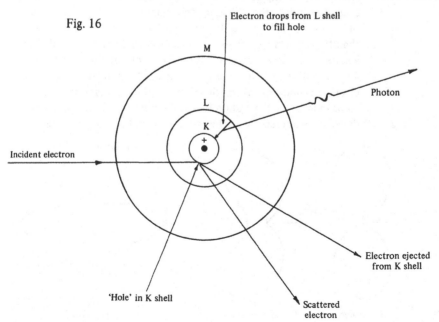

are so severely scattered in matter that the peak is blurred out by the very variable ranges of the individual electrons. Although the specific ionization along the actual path of an individual electron is similar to that of heavy particles, when the ionization produced by a beam of electrons is measured at a particular point in the absorber the total effect is due to a number of electrons moving in different directions with very different energies. The scattering is so severe, especially in the low energy region, that some of the electrons, which have been scattered several times, may in fact be moving backwards. The situation is quite different with a beam of heavy particles. Since they are only slightly scattered the ionization at a particular point is due to a number of particles all of approximately the same energy moving parallel to each other.

The interaction of photons with matter
When measurements are made with a parallel beam of mono-energetic photons from a suitable radioactive source, using the arrangement shown in fig. 9, the intensity of the beam of photons

Fig. 17

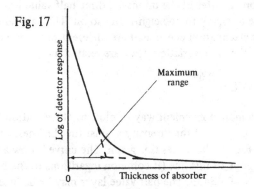

Fig. 18

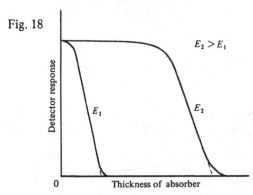

varies with the thickness of the absorber in the manner shown in fig. 19. The intensity of a beam of radiation is measured by the rate of flow of energy per unit area where the measuring area is perpendicular to the direction of flow of the radiation. With monoenergetic photons the intensity is proportional to the number of photons passing through the unit area per unit time. The variation illustrated in fig. 19 is an exponential and the relationship for the intensity of the radiation is

$$I = I_0\, e^{-\mu x}$$

where I is the intensity of the radiation transmitted by a thickness x of the absorber, I_0 being the intensity when the thickness is zero. μ is a constant termed the linear attenuation coefficient; it controls the rate of change of intensity with the thickness of the absorber. Another way of specifying this variation is in terms of the half value layer (HVL). This is the thickness of absorber that exactly halves the intensity of the radiation. As shown in fig. 19, since the intensity varies exponentially, two half value layers transmit one quarter of the intensity, three half value layers reduce the intensity to one eighth and so on. The half value layer and linear attenuation coefficient are different parameters for specifying the same variation; they are related by

$$\mathrm{HVL} = \frac{0.693}{\mu}$$

Often a more convenient way of plotting the variation is to plot the logarithm of the intensity against the thickness of the absorber. Fig. 20 illustrates this graph. The curve is now a straight line. The slope of this line (if common logarithms to the base 10 are used) is -0.4343μ. The half value layer may be deduced by

Fig. 19

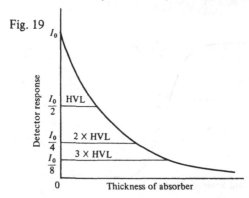

Thickness of absorber

measuring 0.3010 ($\log_{10} 2$) down the $\log_{10} I$ axis from the point where the curve crosses this axis and drawing a line parallel to the thickness axis until it meets the curve.

The reduction of intensity of a beam of photons is quite different from the absorption of charged particles. With a beam of charged particles, as the thickness of the absorber is increased a stage is reached when no particles arrive at the detector since the particles have a finite range. In the case of photons, range is a meaningless term since the probability of a photon being transmitted is finite no matter how thick the absorber is made.

The exponential variation of intensity of the beam originates from the fact that attenuation is an all or none effect. An individual photon is either completely removed from the beam by the absorber or it is not removed at all. This is similar to the disintegration of a radioactive nucleus: the nucleus either disintegrates or remains in its original form, it cannot partly disintegrate. The removal of photons from the beam is due to their interaction with atoms of the absorber. If one considers a thin slab of absorber of thickness δx (fig. 21), the probability of a photon interacting with an atom as it passes through the slab is proportional to the number of atoms in the thickness of the slab and so δI is proportional to δx. Similarly, the probability of removing

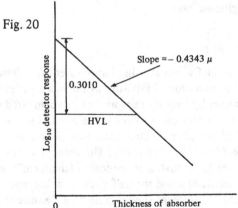

Fig. 20

Slope $= - 0.4343 \mu$

0.3010

HVL

Log$_{10}$ detector response

Thickness of absorber

0

Fig. 21

δx

Intensity I

$I - \delta I$

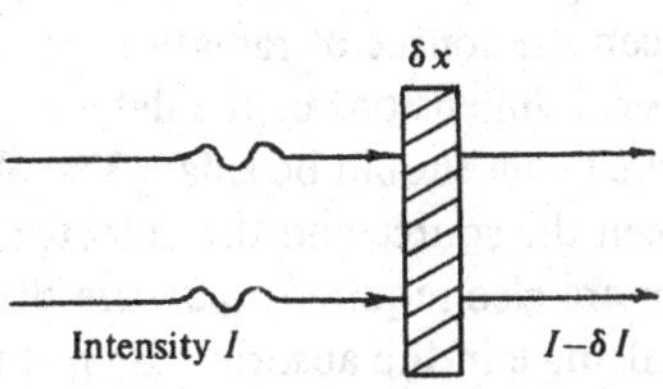

photons from a beam must be proportional to the number of photons entering the slab and so δI is proportional to I. Therefore

$$\delta I \propto I \delta x$$

or

$$\delta I = \mu I \delta x \qquad\qquad (2)$$

where μ is a constant.

In the limiting case where δx is infinitely small

$$dI = -\mu I dx$$

The negative sign is introduced since I decreases as x increases. Integration of this equation yields

$$I = I_0 e^{-\mu x}$$

As we shall see later, when a photon is removed from the beam it need not necessarily disappear but may be scattered at some angle. No matter how small the scattering angle, we consider the photon to have been removed since it is no longer travelling parallel to the incident photons.

Equation 2 is illuminating since it explains the significance of μ. Rearranging we have

$$\mu = \frac{\delta I}{I \delta x}$$

where $\delta I / I$ is the fractional reduction of intensity. Therefore μ is the fractional reduction of intensity of the beam per unit thickness of absorber by very thin absorbers (thin compared with the half value layer). One can also derive the units of μ from this equation. $\delta I / I$ is a plain number since both the top and bottom of the fraction have units of intensity. The units of μ must therefore be the same as $1/\delta x$, that is, reciprocal of length (m^{-1}, cm^{-1}, etc.).

Measurements of μ and the half value layer are made using the experimental arrangement shown in fig. 9. To ensure that the detector is looking at an essentially parallel beam of photons, the distance between the source of radiation and detector should be large, the physical dimensions of the detector should be small and the width of the beam should be small. The absorbers are placed midway between the source and the detector. Small dimensions of the detector are also required to ensure that photons scattered through a small angle in the absorber are not received by the detector. For the same reason the lateral dimensions of the beam are restricted with a suitable diaphragm.

The value of the linear attenuation coefficient, μ, of a beam of photons in an absorbing medium depends on the energy of the photons, the atomic number of the absorber, and the physical state of the absorber. That μ depends on the physical state may be seen by considering a slab of absorber of, say, water, which has a thickness equal to the half value layer. If the water were evaporated to steam, the cross-sectional area remaining constant, the thickness would be greatly increased. The absorber would still contain the same number of atoms and hence the interaction of the beam with it would still be the same. The slab would still reduce the intensity to half its original value, but the thickness (and hence the half value layer) would be greatly increased and so μ would be greatly reduced by the change in state. If μ/ρ is considered instead of μ, where ρ is the density of the absorbing material, this fraction is independent of the physical state since a change in ρ is accompanied by a corresponding change in μ. μ/ρ is termed the mass attenuation coefficient. The dimensions of the mass attenuation coefficient are length^2/mass, since μ has dimensions length^{-1} and the dimensions of ρ are mass/length^3. The units of μ/ρ are m^2 kg^{-1} (or cm^2 g^{-1}). The mass attenuation coefficient measures the fractional reduction of the intensity of the beam per kilogram per square metre by very thin absorbers; it is the fractional reduction of intensity divided by the superficial density (kg m^{-2} or g cm^{-2}) of the absorber.

Measurement of the linear attenuation coefficient involves measuring the linear thickness of the absorber whereas the mass coefficient involves measuring the thickness in terms of the mass per unit area. The thickness could similarly be measured in terms of the number of atoms per unit area, which would yield the atomic attenuation coefficient ($_a\mu$), or the number of electrons per unit area, which would yield the electronic attenuation coefficient ($_e\mu$). These are more fundamental coefficients than the linear or mass coefficients since the interactions of the photons leading to attenuation are either with atoms or individual electrons.

The interaction processes

Various processes may occur when an X-ray photon interacts with matter. These will be considered in order of the energy region in which they are important. At low energies the process of unmodified scattering (Thomson scattering) occurs. In this process the electrons of an atom of the absorber, when subjected to the influence of a photon, oscillate at the same frequency as the photon and re-radiate energy at this frequency. The re-radiated energy will, in general, move in a different direction to the incident photon. The overall effect is that the photon is scattered at some angle to its original direction without a change in wavelength. The process is important only at low energies or for high atomic number absorbers, when the spacing of the electrons in the atom is small compared with the wavelength of the radiation. It is the interaction which is utilized in X-ray diffraction for crystallographic analysis of matter.

In the photoelectric process the incident photon interacts with a bound electron in an atom of the absorber, transferring all of its energy to the electron and ejecting it from the atom. In the Compton process the photon interacts with a 'free' electron, that is, an electron with binding energy small compared with the photon energy. The photon is scattered with reduced energy, the difference between the photon energy before and after the scattering process being imparted to the electron as kinetic energy. At energies above 1.02 MeV the photon may disappear if it enters the field near the nucleus of an atom and all of its energy is converted into the rest mass and kinetic energy of a pair of oppositely charged particles (pair production). At yet higher energies the photon may interact with the nucleus itself causing the ejection of one or more particles. These photodisintegration reactions usually occur at energies of the order of 9 MeV or more. One or two occur at lower energies, the lowest being the photodisintegration of beryllium with a threshold about 1.7 MeV. Photodisintegration reactions can usually be neglected when considering X-ray attenuation since the probability of their occurrence is relatively small.

When a beam of many photons passes through matter all of these attenuation processes may occur simultaneously. The relative importance of each interaction depends on the energy of the photons and the atomic number of the absorbing material. The linear and other attenuation coefficients measure the sum of the effects of the various attenuation processes on the intensity of the beam. The three most important processes are the photoelectric process, the Compton process and pair production, so we can write

$$\mu = \tau + \sigma + \kappa$$

where τ represents the fraction of the total attenuation due to the photoelectric process, σ the fraction due to the Compton process and κ the fraction due to pair production. Similarly, if we are considering the mass attenuation coefficient, we divide this equation throughout by the density, ρ, to give

$$\frac{\mu}{\rho} = \frac{\tau}{\rho} + \frac{\sigma}{\rho} + \frac{\kappa}{\rho}$$

Attenuation and absorption

When a beam of photons passes through matter it is attenuated, that is, photons are removed from the beam and the intensity of the beam is reduced. Some of the energy of photons that have interacted with the matter may be imparted to charged particles. These charged particles may then produce ionization and excitation of the matter as they pass through it. This process, the deposition of energy in the medium, is referred to as absorption. For instance, in the process of unmodified scattering no energy is imparted to the medium and so, although the beam is attenuated, no absorption occurs. In each of the three main interaction processes energetic charged particles are produced and absorption of energy in the medium follows the removal of photons from the beam.

It is unfortunate that the term absorption has been, in the past, and indeed still is, loosely used to describe attenuation rather than true absorption. The true absorption is described by a separate coefficient, μ_{en}, the absorption coefficient. In all three of the main interaction processes only part of the energy of the incident photon is transferred to a charged particle and deposited in the medium. The rest of the energy is in the form of one or more photons and this energy is not necessarily deposited in the medium near the site of the primary interaction. The attenuation coefficient μ is divided into two parts: μ_{en}, which represents the energy transferred to charged particles, and μ_s, which represents the energy which appears as photons. μ_{en} is defined as the fraction of the original photon energy transferred to charged particles and μ_s the fraction of the photon energy which is scattered. This definition of μ_{en} is, in fact, slightly erroneous since some of the energy of charged particles may be lost from the medium as bremsstrahlung. Bremsstrahlung loss is usually small though, particularly in low atomic number media, and becomes significant only at high energies.

With these definitions of μ_{en} and μ_s we have

$$\mu = \mu_{en} + \mu_s$$

and similarly

$$\mu/\rho = \mu_{en}/\rho + \mu_s/\rho$$

The attenuation coefficients τ, σ and κ for the individual processes can similarly be split into absorption and scatter components.

The photoelectric process
In the photoelectric process a photon with energy greater than the binding energy of one of the electrons in an atom imparts all of its energy to this electron. The photon disappears and the electron gains kinetic energy given by

$$E = h\nu - E_B$$

where E is the kinetic energy of the electron, $h\nu$ the energy of the photon and E_B the binding energy of the electron in the atom. The electron, which is ejected from the atom, is referred to as a photoelectron. The process is illustrated in fig. 22 where the photon interacts with a K electron. The ejection of the photoelectron leaves a hole in the shell and this is then filled by an electron dropping in from an outer shell. Since the outer electrons are less tightly bound to the nucleus, surplus energy is radiated as characteristic radiation during the transition.

The variation of τ, the photoelectric attenuation coefficient, with photon energy is shown in fig. 23. At low energies the photon has sufficient energy to eject electrons only from the outer shells.

Fig. 22

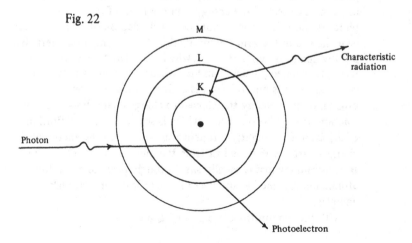

As the photon energy is increased a series of discontinuities appears and there are sudden increases in the attenuation coefficient. These discontinuities occur when the photon has sufficient energy to eject electrons from the different L subshells. The discontinuities are referred to as the L absorption edges. At these edges the energy of the photon is just equal to the binding energy of the L electrons. At energies above the L edges attenuation occurs in the L shell and the M shell etc. With further increase of photon energy yet another discontinuity appears. This is the K edge and occurs when the photon has sufficient energy to eject electrons from the K shell. Above the K edge attenuation takes place in all the shells of the atom. In the energy region above the K edge most of the attenuation occurs in the K shell, and the contribution from the L and other shells is relatively small. Similarly, in the region between the K and L edges the contribution from the L shell is much larger than that due to the M and outer shells. The energies at which the edges occur depend on the atomic number of the absorber. The K edge of lead is at about 88 keV whereas in oxygen the K edge occurs at about 530 eV. Away from the absorption edges the linear attenuation coefficient, τ, and the mass attenuation coefficient, τ/ρ, are approximately inversely proportional to the photon energy cubed, i.e. τ and τ/ρ are approximately proportional to λ^3, where λ is the wavelength of the radiation. The value of τ also varies approximately as Z^4 where Z is the atomic number of the absorber. Since the density of most solids is roughly proportional to Z, the mass attenuation coefficient (τ/ρ) is approximately proportional to Z^3. It is evident from these variations that attenuation by the photo-

Fig. 23

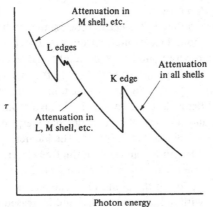

Photon energy

electric process is important at low energies and for high atomic number absorbers.

The angular distribution of the photoelectrons produced in the process is rather similar to the bremsstrahlung distributions given in fig. 15. At low energies they are produced predominantly at right angles to the direction of motion of the photons. With an increase in energy the lobes swing forward in the same direction as the motion of the photon.

As we have already seen, in the photoelectric process the energy given to the photoelectron as kinetic energy is equal to $h\nu - E_B$, where $h\nu$ is the energy of the photon and E_B is the binding energy of the electron. The energy which is subsequently radiated as one or more photons of characteristic radiation is equal to E_B. As we have also seen, for high atomic number materials E_B may be large and the characteristic radiation produced may be penetrating; consequently its energy may be lost from the absorber. In the case of low atomic number materials such as air, water and soft tissue, i.e. the materials of main biological interest, the highest value of E_B is due to the K shell of oxygen and has a value of 530 eV. The characteristic radiation due to photoelectric attenuation in oxygen is of very low energy and readily interacts with atoms near the site where it is produced. The energy of these photons is thus rapidly degraded to the motion of electrons of the absorber near the site where the original interaction occurred. Thus, virtually all of the original photon energy is deposited in the absorbing medium close to the site of the original interaction and τ_{en} is equal to τ for these low atomic number absorbers.

The Compton process
In contrast to the photoelectric process, in which the photon interacts with a bound electron, the Compton process takes place with a 'free' or loosely bound electron, that is, an electron with binding energy small compared with the photon energy. This condition usually prevails in low atomic number materials such as air, water and tissue, but not necessarily in high atomic number materials, in which the electrons may have large binding energies. The process is illustrated in fig. 24. The incident photon of energy $h\nu$ and wavelength λ collides with the free electron and imparts some of its energy to it. The electron recoils at an angle θ to the original direction of the photon and the photon is scattered through an angle ϕ with reduced energy $h\nu'$ and increased wavelength λ'.

The process is somewhat similar to the collision between a moving billiard ball and one at rest. In the billiard ball collision, if the collision is head-on the moving ball transfers all of its energy to the stationary ball and this ball then moves in the same direction as the other was moving before the collision. If the collision is glancing, the stationary ball acquires very little energy and tends to move at right angles to the original path of the moving ball; the moving ball is deflected through a small angle during the collision. When a photon collides with a free electron the value of θ lies between zero and 90° and the recoil electron always has a component of velocity in the same direction as the original photon. The value of ϕ can lie anywhere between zero and 180°. θ and ϕ are related to each other and, in general, the greater the value of ϕ, the smaller is θ and the greater the fraction of the energy of the incident photon that is transferred to the recoil electron.

The change of wavelength of the photon during the process is given by

$$\lambda' - \lambda = 2.42 \times 10^{-12} \, (1 - \cos \phi) \text{ metres}$$

or

$$\Delta\lambda = 0.00242 \, (1 - \cos \phi) \text{ nanometres (nm)}$$

The expression is independent of the energy of the photon and increases with ϕ, being zero when $\phi = 0$ and a maximum when $\phi = 180°$. For a particular energy of the incident photon the maximum energy transfer to the electron occurs when the photon is scattered backwards. Under these circumstances $\Delta\lambda = 0.0048$ nm. Clearly this change in the photon wavelength will have

Fig. 24

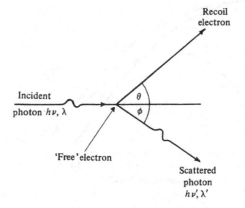

negligible effect on the photon energy at long wavelengths but will cause a large change of energy at short wavelengths. For example, if the incident photon wavelength is 0.1 nm, corresponding to a photon energy of 12 keV, the back scattered photon has a wavelength of 0.1048 nm which corresponds to a five per cent change of photon energy. This fraction of the photon energy is transferred to the recoil electron. If the wavelength of the incident photon is 0.0001 nm, corresponding to an energy of 12 MeV, the back scattered photon has a wavelength of 0.0049 nm, which corresponds to a decrease in photon energy to about 250 keV. The recoil electron thus acquires 11.75 MeV, or roughly ninety-seven per cent of the original photon energy. These are two extreme cases, where the photon is scattered backwards, but two important features will be noted. In general, the fraction of the energy of the incident photon which is transferred to the recoil electron increases with the photon energy and the scattered radiation is always of lower energy than the incident radiation; this is particularly so for high energy radiation and large scattering angles.

   The attenuation coefficient, σ, for the Compton process is a complicated function of the photon energy. The variation of σ with photon energy is shown in fig. 25. It is a continuously decreasing function of the photon energy. Since the Compton process takes place with essentially free electrons, the attenuation coefficient per electron ($e\sigma$) is independent of the atomic number of the material. It is the electronic coefficient, $e\sigma$, which is plotted in fig. 25. The Compton coefficient, σ, consists of two components, one, σ_s, representing the scattered energy and the

Fig. 25

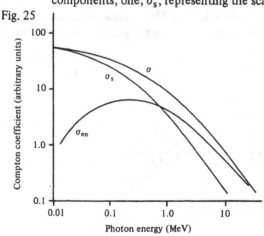

other, σ_{en}, representing the absorbed energy, where $\sigma = \sigma_s + \sigma_{en}$. The general forms of σ_s and σ_{en} are also indicated in fig. 25. At low photon energies, although σ is large σ_{en} is small, because relatively little energy is transferred to the recoil electron. With increasing photon energy σ_{en} increases, passing through a broad maximum at about 500 keV and tending towards the value of σ at high energies because the fraction of the photon energy transferred to the recoil electron tends to unity at high energies. Thus at low photon energies, in the Compton process, most of the energy of the photon is scattered, whereas at high energies most of it is absorbed.

The angle of ejection of the recoil electron is never greater than $90°$. The average angle decreases as the photon energy increases until at high energies the average angle is small and the most probable direction of motion of the electron is in the same direction as the incident photon. At low energies the scattered photon is equally likely to be scattered forwards or backwards. The probability of being scattered forwards increases with the incident photon energy until at high energies the forward direction is the most probable direction. The predominantly forward direction of the recoil electron and the scattered photon at high energies leads to the effect called 'build-up' when an extended medium is irradiated with a beam of high energy photons.

Since the Compton coefficient per electron, $e\sigma$, is independent of the atomic number of the absorber and since nearly all materials contain the same number of electrons per unit mass, the mass attenuation coefficient, σ/ρ, is approximately independent of the atomic number. The exception to this generalization is hydrogen, which contains twice as many electrons per unit mass as other materials. Hydrogenous materials show an enhanced attenuation from the Compton process. With the exception of hydrogenous materials, since σ/ρ is approximately independent of Z and since ρ is approximately proportional to Z, σ is approximately proportional to Z.

Pair production

The process of pair production is illustrated in fig. 26. In this process a high energy photon enters the field near the nucleus of the atom and interacts with the field. The energy of the photon is converted into the rest energy and kinetic energy of two oppositely charged particles, an electron–positron pair. Charge is conserved during the collision since the charge on the electron is equal in magnitude to that on the positron. The presence of the nucleus is necessary during the process in order that momentum may be conserved; the process cannot take place in free space. The nucleus recoils with some momentum and consequently acquires some of the energy of the original photon, but owing to the high mass of the nucleus the amount of energy it receives is insignificant compared with the energy of the electron—positron pair.

The interaction has an energy threshold equal to the energy-equivalent of the rest masses of the two particles created. The energy-equivalent of a mass M is Mc^2 where c is the velocity of light. The masses of the electron and positron are each equal to 9.11×10^{-31} kg and since the velocity of light is equal to 3×10^8 m s^{-1}, the energy equivalent of the two masses is $2 \times (9.11 \times 10^{-31}) \times (3 \times 10^8)^2$, which is equal to 1.64×10^{-13} J. Since 1 MeV is equivalent to 1.6×10^{-13} J, the masses are equivalent to 1.02 MeV and the interaction cannot occur with photons of energy lower than this value. If the photon producing the pair has energy greater than this threshold, the surplus energy is shared between the two particles. In general the particles do not have equal energy but their total kinetic energy is related to the photon energy by the equation

$$E_{el} + E_{pos} = h\nu - 1.02 \text{ MeV}$$

where E_{el} is the kinetic energy of the electron and E_{pos} is that of the positron.

Fig. 26

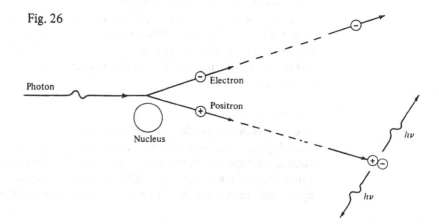

Subsequent to formation, the electron moves through the matter dissipating its kinetic energy by ionization and excitation until it is eventually brought to rest. The electron maintains its identity after it has come to rest, eventually combining with a positive ion to form a neutral atom. The positron, on the other hand, has but a transitory existence in matter. From the instant of its creation it is vulnerable to annihilation by combining with an electron from the matter in the reaction

$$e^+ + e^- \longrightarrow \text{Energy}$$

The mutual annihilation of a positron and an electron can take place at any energy of the positron; there is, however, a greater probability that annihilation will take place when the positron has been brought to rest by losing its energy by ionization and excitation. The usual product of annihilation is two photons each of energy 0.51 MeV moving in opposite directions. If the positron is annihilated before it is brought to rest its kinetic energy is also given to the photons, but in this case the photons do not travel in opposite directions.

The variation with energy of κ, the component of the linear attenuation coefficient due to pair production, is a complex function. It is zero below 1.02 MeV and increases with energy above this value, in contrast with τ and σ, both of which decrease with increasing energy. κ is approximately proportional to Z^2 where Z is the atomic number of the absorber. κ/ρ, the mass attenuation coefficient, is approximately proportional to Z.

The relationship between κ and the absorption coefficient κ_{en} may be deduced by considering the fraction of the original photon energy that is dissipated as ionization and excitation. If the energy of the incident photon is $h\nu$, then, neglecting any energy lost by the electron–positron pair as bremsstrahlung, and assuming that the positron is brought to rest before it is annihilated, the energy that is truly absorbed in the medium is $h\nu - 1.02$ MeV. Therefore the fraction of the energy of the incident photon that is absorbed is $(h\nu - 1.02)/h\nu$
and

$$\kappa_{en} = \frac{(h\nu - 1.02)\kappa}{h\nu}$$

κ_{en} is considerably smaller than κ if the photon energy is not very much greater than the threshold, but tends towards κ at high photon energies.

The total attenuation coefficient

The total attenuation coefficients μ and μ/ρ are the sum of the coefficients of the three main processes.

Mass attenuation coefficients of water, copper and lead, being representative of low, medium and high atomic number materials, are illustrated in figs. 27, 28 and 29 as functions of photon energy. In these diagrams logarithmic scales are used for both axes to encompass the wide range of the variables. The mass coefficients for the individual interactions are plotted, together with the sum of their effects. Included in the graphs are the attenuation coefficients for unmodified scattering. A number of important features will be noted.

(i)   In each of the curves of μ/ρ the main contribution at low energies is due to the photoelectric process. This is followed by a region in

Fig. 27

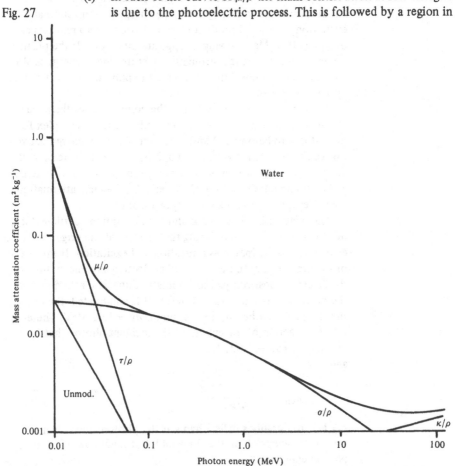

which the Compton process is the dominant factor and at high
energies pair production is the most important interaction.

(ii)   In the energy range considered (not lower than 10 keV) unmodified scattering is relatively unimportant. It is greatest for lead and
at low energies is greater than the Compton coefficient but is less
than the photoelectric coefficient. In lead it becomes significant
only in the region just below the K absorption edge.

(iii)   The variation of the photoelectric coefficient with energy appears
as straight lines on these graphs due to the logarithmic scales.
While the K and L edges of lead appear, those of copper and water

Fig. 28

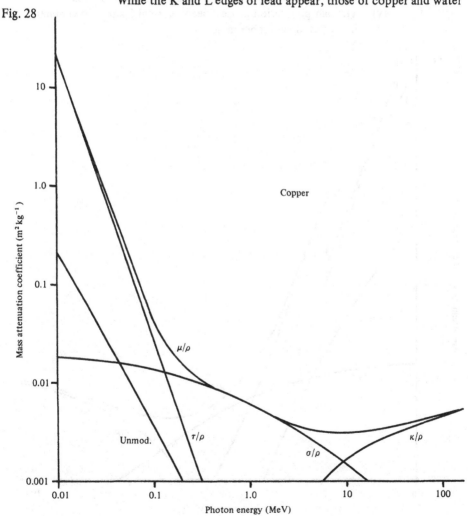

are not seen owing to the low energies at which their K edges occur (copper 8.99 keV, oxygen 0.53 keV). The marked increase of the photoelectric process with atomic number will be noted as will the greater energy range over which it contributes significantly to the total attenuation in high atomic number materials.

(iv) The curves of σ/ρ for copper and lead are approximately the same, whereas that for water is rather greater owing to its hydrogen content. Over a wide range of energies, from about 60 keV to about 5 MeV, the attenuation in water and materials of similar composition is almost entirely due to the Compton process.

(v) The pair production process becomes significant at lower energies in high atomic number materials.

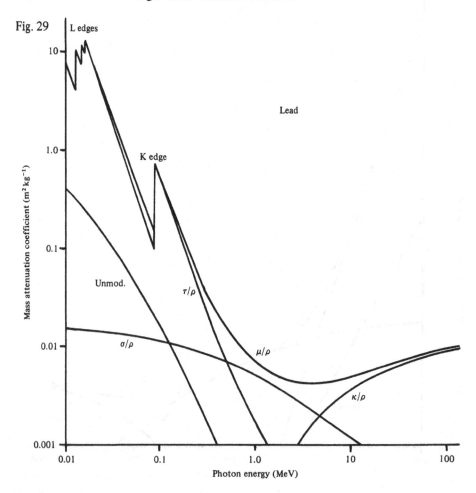

Fig. 29

(vi) Each of the curves of μ/ρ shows a minimum owing to the decrease of τ/ρ and σ/ρ and the increase of κ/ρ with energy. This minimum occurs at lower energies in high atomic number materials. In lead it occurs at 4 MeV, in copper at 8 MeV and in water at about 50 MeV.

(vii) The curves are plotted for monoenergetic photons. The attenuation coefficient obtained with a heterogeneous beam of X-rays, produced by the bremsstrahlung process, is an average over the range of photon energies of the beam.

Secondary electrons
The charged particles produced in the three main interactions – photoelectrons, recoil electrons and electron–positron pairs – are given the collective name of secondary electrons. When a beam of photons interacts with matter, the secondary electrons produced have a range of energies from near zero up to a maximum value, depending on the photon energy. The secondary electrons deposit their kinetic energy by excitation and ionization in the surrounding medium. Thus, energy which is removed from the photon beam is deposited in the absorbing medium by way of the interaction of the secondary electrons. The factors which affect the deposition of energy in the medium (chiefly photon energy and atomic number of the medium) exert their influence in the production of secondary electrons in the three interaction processes.

The interaction of neutrons with matter
The interaction of a beam of neutrons with matter is quite different from that of either charged particles or photons. Charged particles ionize and excite directly, owing to the interaction of their charge with electrons in the medium. Neutrons have no charge and the ionization and excitation they produce is by secondary effects resulting from their interaction with nuclei. In this respect their behaviour is similar to that of photons, but while photons interact with the atomic electrons or the field around the nucleus, neutrons interact with the nucleus itself. Three types of interaction can occur: the neutron may be captured by the nucleus and the resulting nucleus may emit one or more particles (including photons); the neutron may be scattered inelastically by the nucleus; or, finally, the neutron may be scattered elastically.

Neutron capture
Most nuclei show a relatively high probability for absorption of

neutrons at some neutron energy. Since the resulting nucleus is usually in an excited state and returns to its ground state by emitting the surplus energy as a photon, the process is known as a (n, γ) reaction, or radiative capture. The product nucleus may be radioactive and undergo subsequent disintegration. The probability of the capture reaction occurring varies inversely with the neutron velocity and so is more important at low neutron energies. If the energy of the neutron is sufficiently high it is possible for the nucleus to emit a charged particle such as a proton or alpha particle. Reactions of this type have threshold energies below which they do not occur. In a few high atomic number materials the nucleus may undergo fission subsequent to capture, breaking into two relatively large fragments.

Inelastic scattering

In this type of collision the neutron transfers some of its energy to the nucleus as excitation energy. The nucleus gains no kinetic energy but is raised to an excited level in a similar fashion to the excitation of an atom. The nucleus returns to its ground state by the emission of a photon. This type of collision also has a threshold, depending on the excitation energies of the nucleus. Inelastic scattering by medium and heavy nuclei is important for neutrons with energies above 1 MeV but is practically negligible at lower energies.

Elastic scattering

In the elastic scattering collision the neutron transfers kinetic energy to the nucleus. The nucleus recoils from the collision and, since it is a charged particle, dissipates its kinetic energy by ionization and excitation of the atoms of the surrounding medium. During the collision both momentum and kinetic energy are conserved.

A rigorous treatment of the energy loss of a beam of fast neutrons by elastic scattering in an extended medium is mathematically complicated but the physical processes involved are quite simple and the most useful results are easily derived by treating the collision as if it occurred between two billiard balls of different mass, one of which is at rest. The collision is illustrated in fig. 30. The neutron of mass m, velocity v_0 and energy E_0 collides with a stationary nucleus of mass M. After the collision the neutron moves at an angle θ to its original direction with a velocity v and energy E. The recoil nucleus acquires energy equal to $E_0 - E$ and moves at an angle ϕ to the original direction of the neutron. The energy of the recoil nucleus is given by

$$E_0 - E = \frac{4\,M}{(M + m)^2} \, (E_0 \cos^2 \phi)$$

This expression tends to zero as M becomes large, showing that high atomic number materials are not very effective at slowing neutrons. For head-on collisions $\phi = 0$ and the expression for the energy of the recoil nucleus reduces to

$$E_0 - E = \frac{4\,M\,E_0}{(M + m)^2}$$

As an example, if carbon is the slowing material $M \sim 12\,m$ and twenty-eight per cent of the neutron energy is transferred to the recoil nucleus. If the slowing material is hydrogen $M \sim m$ and $E_0 - E = E_0$, i.e. all of the energy of the neutron is transferred to the hydrogen nucleus in a head-on collision and the neutron is brought to rest. For glancing collisions $\phi \sim 90°$ and the expression for the energy of the recoil nucleus reduces to zero.

In a particular collision ϕ may have any value between $90°$ and zero and the energy of the recoil nucleus may have any value between zero and the maximum possible, depending on its mass. The value of ϕ depends on the angle between the initial direction of motion of the neutron and the line between the centres of the particles at the instant of contact. All values of this angle between zero (head-on collision) and $90°$ (glancing collision) are possible. To determine the average fraction of the energy lost by a neutron in a single collision the expression for $(E_0 - E)/E_0$ must be suitably averaged over all possible values of ϕ.

When a neutron enters an extended medium it will lose this average fraction of its energy at each collision, its energy gradually being reduced until, eventually, it is of the same order as the thermal energies (0.025 eV) of the nuclei of the medium.

Fig. 30

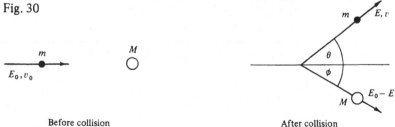

Before collision   After collision

Table 1 lists the average number of collisions required to reduce the energy of neutrons from 10 MeV to thermal energies for a few representative nuclei. It will be noticed that hydrogen is very effective at slowing neutrons because its nucleus has approximately the same mass as the neutron, whereas uranium, with a much heavier nucleus, is ineffective. In the case of hydrogen, neglecting the small mass difference between the proton and neutron, the neutron loses on average thirty-seven per cent of its energy at each collision.

When a beam of fast neutrons enters an extended medium the three interaction processes — neutron capture, inelastic scattering and elastic scattering — compete with each other. Which of the processes predominates depends on the nature of the medium and the energy of the neutrons. If the medium is tissue, almost two-thirds of the nuclei are protons and elastic scattering by these nuclei is the predominant interaction. Although the other nuclei, such as oxygen and carbon, also scatter elastically, the average amount of energy transferred in these collisions is much less than is transferred in a collision with a hydrogen nucleus. Neutron capture does occur in tissue, the main reactions being $H(n, \gamma)D$ and $^{14}N(n, p)^{14}C$, but the probability of these reactions occurring is very much less than the probability of elastic scattering by hydrogen.

Table 1. *The average number of collisions required to reduce the energy of neutrons from 10 MeV to thermal energies in some representative materials*

Nuclei	Mass relative to neutron	Average number of collisions from 10 MeV to 0.025 eV
Hydrogen	1	20
Deuterium	2	27
Carbon	12	125
Nitrogen	14	145
Oxygen	16	165
Uranium	238	2360

3. The effects of ionizing radiation on matter in bulk

So far we have dealt with the interaction of ionizing radiation (charged particles, photons and neutrons) with matter at the atomic level and seen that the radiations are capable of ionizing and exciting atoms. The energy deposited in an extended medium by ionization and excitation may produce effects in the medium which are transitory, such as the heating effect, or more or less permanent, such as the latent image formed in a photographic emulsion. The exact nature of the effects which follow the initial interaction of the primary radiation depends on the characteristics of the particular medium.

The train of events which occurs when primary ionizing radiation enters an absorbing medium is shown in fig. 31. If the primary radiation is a charged particle, such as an alpha particle or beta ray, the events follow the upper branch. If the primary radiation is a photon, it interacts with an atom by the photoelectric process, Compton process or pair production to produce a secondary electron, which follows the upper branch, and a photon, which follows the lower branch. This scattered photon may interact further with the medium to produce more secondary electrons. If the primary radiation is a neutron, the charged particle is a

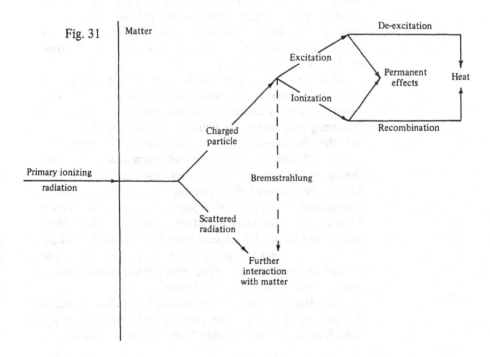

Fig. 31

recoil nucleus and the scattered particle is the neutron itself, with reduced energy, which also interacts further with the medium.

In the upper branch of the diagram the charged particle produces excitation and ionization. Excited atoms return to their ground state with the emission of their excitation energy as photons, mainly in the visible and ultraviolet part of the spectrum. Most of this energy is gradually degraded by further atomic and molecular excitations until it appears as thermal energy of the medium. A small part of the excitation energy in the medium may produce permanent effects. Similarly, the ions produced by the charged particle recombine and most of the energy required to form them appears as thermal energy. A small part of the total energy dissipated as ionization by the charged particle may also produce permanent effects. Thus, most of the energy of the charged particle appears promptly as thermal energy of the medium, and only a very small fraction, at the most of the order of a few per cent, may be trapped by the production of permanent effects.

The term permanent is used in a relative sense rather than absolutely. The thermal energy appears very quickly after the passage of the particle and may be lost fairly quickly from the medium by conduction, convection and radiation. The disappearance of the initial ionization is even quicker. The permanent effects may also vanish with time, but in this case the time involved is very much longer.

All of the effects in matter in bulk are, or have been at some time, used to measure amounts of ionizing radiation. Transitory effects, such as ionization, are useful since they are adaptable to measuring both amounts of radiation and the rate of flow of the radiation. Permanent effects are most easily used to measure quantity of radiation and are less readily adapted to measuring the rate at which the radiation arrives. They are useful in that they not only have a built-in integrating effect but may also give a permanent record of the radiation. Since transitory effects can be used to measure the rate at which the radiation flows, they can be used for making measurements during the course of an irradiation, whereas the permanent effects can only be used to measure the total amount of radiation and have to be evaluated after the termination of the irradiation.

If an effect of the radiation in matter is to be used to measure the quantity of radiation, one criterion that it must satisfy is that the effect must be reproducible. Many effects are produced by ionizing radiations in biological systems, but biological materials generally show a wide variability in their characteristics and are not used as precision dosemeters. For this reason biological effects will not be described here.

The following description of the effects produced by ionizing radiation in matter in bulk does not pretend to be comprehensive. It is intended as an introduction to the main effects used for measurement purposes.

Transitory effects
Ionization in gases
When ionization is produced in a medium, the ions are always produced in pairs. For every positive ion produced there is a negative ion, which is usually an electron, since the original matter was neutral and charge is conserved. Ionization in solids and liquids is relatively difficult to demonstrate whereas in gases the effect can easily be shown using the experimental arrangement of fig. 32. In this diagram P_1 and P_2 are two parallel conducting plates separated by a space filled with a gas, such as air. B is a battery which can be tapped to provide different potential differences between P_1 and P_2, and A is a sensitive current meter. In the absence of ionizing radiation the meter indicates zero current owing to the good insulating properties of air. When the air between P_1 and P_2 is irradiated with X-rays the meter shows a deflection, demonstrating that the air has become conducting under the influence of the X-rays.

If the intensity of the X-rays is kept constant and the potential difference between P_1 and P_2 is varied, by altering the tapping of the battery, the reading of the meter varies as shown in fig. 33. With zero potential difference between P_1 and P_2 all of the ions produced in the air recombine. There is a natural tendency for this to happen owing to the Coulomb attraction of the opposite charges on the ions. An individual ion may not necessarily recombine with its original partner, but combines with whichever oppositely charged ion happens to exert the greatest attraction on

Fig. 32

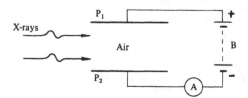

it. As the collecting voltage is increased the ions move under the influence of the electric field between the plates. The negative ions drift towards the positive plate (P_1) and the positive ions drift towards the negative plate (P_2). The applied field may exert a greater influence on individual ions than the field due to any of their neighbours and so they drift along the lines of force until they arrive at the plates. The negative ions may be either free electrons or neutral molecules which have temporarily acquired a free electron. In either case, on arrival at P_1 the electron is driven round the circuit by the battery until it arrives at P_2 where it neutralizes a positive ion. The current indicated by the meter is due to the negatively charged ions produced in the air between the plates. The positive ions do not travel in the external circuit through A and B owing to their much greater dimensions.

With small collecting fields many of the ions experience a force from their oppositely charged neighbours which is greater than the force due to the collecting field and consequently combine with them. As the collecting field is increased, less recombination occurs and the current indicated by the meter increases. The increase of meter reading with collecting voltage continues until, eventually, no recombination occurs and all of the ions are extracted by the collecting field. This condition is indicated by the plateau in fig. 33. The value of the ionization current when this condition prevails is termed the saturation current.

The ease of collecting ions in gases compared with solids and liquids originates in the greater molecular spacing in the gas phase. The effect is twofold: it is partly because the ions can travel farther apart when they are first formed, before they are slowed down by collisions with molecules of the gas, and partly because

Fig. 33

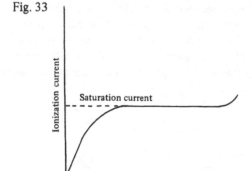

Saturation current

Ionization current

0   Potential difference between P_1 and P_2

the greater separation of the molecules allows the ions to acquire greater velocities under the influence of the applied field.

The negative ions produced initially by the ionizing particles are electrons and these show much greater mobility under the influence of a field than the positive ions, owing to their very much smaller mass. In some gases, such as oxygen, the neutral molecules show an affinity for free electrons, the electron tending to attach itself loosely to the molecule to make a negative ion. This type of negative ion has a mobility of the same order as positive ions. Gases which show this characteristic are termed electronegative gases.

If the electric field applied to an ionized gas containing free electrons is increased to a high value, another effect takes place. The current increases above the plateau value. A free electron collides with many neutral gas molecules during its passage to the positive electrode. In the interval between collisions the electron is accelerated by the field and gains kinetic energy. Provided that the electric intensity is not too great and that the average distance between collisions is small, the electron does not gain sufficient energy to produce ionization of the molecules when it collides with them. It transfers its energy to them as excitation energy. But if either the electric intensity is increased or the pressure of the gas is reduced, the amount of kinetic energy the electron gains between collisions may exceed the energy needed to ionize a gas molecule. In these circumstances, when the electron collides with a neutral molecule it may ionize it, producing a positive ion and another free electron. This free electron is also accelerated by the field and the two electrons may each produce ionization when they next collide, yielding a total of four electrons, and so on. This effect is known as gas multiplication. It is utilized in the Geiger–Müller counter to detect individual ionizing particles such as beta rays. The effect, which is indicated by the rise at the end of the plateau of fig. 33, should be avoided in ionization chambers since it leads to a spurious value of the ionization current.

The average amount of energy required to form an ion pair in a gas, usually given the symbol $\overline{W}$, may also be measured with the apparatus shown in fig. 32. If the beam of X-rays is replaced by a beam of monoenergetic electrons of known energy and the length of the plates is made greater than the range of the electrons in the gas, the electrons will expend all their energy between the plates, ionizing and exciting the gas molecules. The total number of ion pairs formed is determined from the current in the external circuit (the apparatus must be operated under conditions where recombination and gas multiplication do not occur). The total amount of energy required to form this number of ion pairs is determined from the energy of the incident electrons and the number of them entering the gas. The ratio of this amount of energy to the number of ion pairs formed gives the average value of the energy required to produce one ion pair. Similar methods are used to determine the value of $\overline{W}$ for other directly ionizing particles and for indirectly ionizing radiation.

Values of $\overline{W}$ determined by these methods show that the average energy required to form an ion pair is more or less independent of the nature of the radiation producing the ionization and of its energy. And they vary surprisingly little with the gas in which the ionization is produced. In air, the gas most frequently used in ionization chambers, the value of $\overline{W}$ is about 33.7 eV per ion pair and, when measured for electrons or photons, is believed to be independent of their energy. This value of $\overline{W}$ is considerably in excess of the ionization potentials of the constituent molecules of air. The ionization potential (a misnomer since it is an energy, not a potential) is the least amount of energy required to remove an electron from a free, unexcited atom. The ionization potentials of both oxygen and nitrogen are about 14 eV. The difference between the value of $\overline{W}$ and the ionization potential is due to excitation of air molecules.

Ionization in gases, particularly air, is an important effect for measuring ionizing radiation since it leads to a very flexible technique. The ionization current may easily be altered by changing the volume of gas irradiated and the current flowing in the external circuit of the ion chamber may be amplified by electronic techniques to give a wide range of sensitivities. Furthermore, the ionization current is proportional to the rate at which ions are produced in the gas, which is proportional to the rate of arrival of the ionizing particles at the gas volume. Integration of the current, by allowing it to charge a capacitor, gives the total charge liberated by the radiation, which is proportional to the total number of particles entering the chamber. Thus ionization measurements can be used to measure both the intensity of the radiation and the total amount of radiation in a given time.

The heating effect

Referring to fig. 31 it will be seen that virtually all of the energy of the incident particles eventually appears as thermal energy of the absorbing medium. This increase of thermal energy changes the temperature of the medium and, although the temperature change is usually small, it may be measured accurately with modern techniques. If the change of temperature is measured and the heat capacity of the medium is known the amount of energy deposited in the medium may be determined. The advantage of using this effect for measuring radiation is that, provided a medium is chosen in which permanent effects are not produced, all of the energy deposited by the radiation appears as thermal energy and so this method is an absolute method of measuring energy deposited by the radiation, since it depends on the measurement of only two fundamental quantities. The disadvantage of the technique is that it is relatively insensitive owing to the small change of temperature produced by the radiation. The effect lends itself to the measurement of the total amount of energy deposited by the radiation, rather than the rate at which the energy is deposited.

The fluorescent effect

A number of materials, such as zinc sulphide, calcium tungstate and some plastics, have the property of emitting visible light while they are being irradiated with ionizing radiations. This effect is utilized in the intensifying screens used in diagnostic radiology to reduce the exposure time required to take X-ray pictures. It is also used in the phosphor of a scintillation counter. The effect is not used very much in radiation dosimetry since the quantity of light produced is very dependent on small amounts of impurity in the material and may be very dependent on the energy of the radiation.

The effect on electrical conductivity

When ionizing radiation is absorbed in a solid body the charged particles (primary radiation, secondary electrons or recoil nuclei) produce ionization and excitation of the atoms of the body as they traverse it. The presence of the ions might be expected to influence the electrical conductivity of the material. In good conductors, such as metals, the change of conductivity is usually negligible, but in the case of semiconductors and insulators the change may be pronounced and may be readily measured by attaching electrodes to the body. In many instances the change of conductivity is transitory and measurement of the change can be used to determine the intensity of the radiation. In some cases the change is permanent and can be used to determine the total amount of radiation received by the body.

Typical examples of materials which are used to measure ionizing radiation by utilizing this effect are p–n junctions of silicon (often lithium-drifted), of germanium and of gallium arsenide. The devices behave, in effect, as solid state ionization chambers, but they usually have much higher sensitivity than the common air-filled chamber. The enhanced sensitivity originates from two sources. In the first place, the density of the semiconductors is of the order of two thousand times that of air at atmospheric pressure owing to the atoms being packed much closer together and so, when irradiated with X-rays, photons have a two thousand times greater probability of interacting and producing secondary electrons than in the same volume of air. In the second place, the average energy required to produce an ion pair in a semiconductor is of the order of ten times less than in air and so a charged particle of a given energy can produce about ten times as many ions in a semiconductor as in air. Thus one would expect the response of a semiconducting device to be of the order of twenty thousand times greater than that of an air-filled chamber of the same volume when they are irradiated with X-rays.

In another class of similar materials, examples of which are cadmium sulphide and cadmium selenide and a number of organic insulators, such as polyethylene and anthracene, the detector behaves as though it has an internal amplifier and even greater sensitivities are obtained.

Permanent effects
Thermoluminescence
A number of materials, notably lithium fluoride and lithium borate, emit light when they are heated subsequent to irradiation with ionizing radiations. During the irradiation, electrons are produced by the ionization process and some of these free electrons are trapped by trapping centres in the crystal lattice. On heating to a suitable temperature the electrons are freed from the traps and emit energy as light. Although the amount of light emitted is small it can be measured with a photomultiplier tube. Since the material has to be heated after the irradiation, this effect is applicable only to measuring amounts of radiation rather than its intensity. The effect has been developed into a dosemeter with a wide range of sensitivities.

The photographic effect

When a photographic emulsion is exposed to ionizing radiations a latent image is formed in the emulsion in a similar fashion to that formed when the emulsion is exposed to visible light. The emulsion consists of small crystals of silver halide suspended in gelatine. During exposure those crystals which are traversed by charged particles are rendered developable, and if the emulsion is subsequently treated with a suitable solution of reducing agents the developable crystals are reduced to metallic silver, giving a visible image. The amount of blackening produced by the metallic silver is correlated with the amount of radiation the emulsion received. Unfortunately the blackening of the emulsion is sensitive to the energy of the radiation producing it. For this reason photographic emulsions are not used extensively in dosimetry except in personnel monitoring where a high degree of accuracy is not required. If the developed emulsion is viewed with a microscope it is possible to see the actual tracks of charged particles. This technique has been used extensively in nuclear physics and cosmic ray physics. The photographic effect is also used in the autoradiographic technique to show the distribution of radioactive materials in biological specimens.

The chemical effect

The joining together of atoms in molecules and the reactions between molecules are affected by the outer valence electrons. These electrons are only loosely bound to the nucleus, their energies being of the order of a few electron volts. Factors which influence the energy of these outer electrons, such as irradiation with ionizing particles, may be expected to modify the way in which the molecules react and one might expect different reactions to occur under the influence of such stimuli than normally occur.

Some of the effects produced may be of a transitory nature but, depending on the material irradiated, permanent effects may also be produced. An example of the chemical effect of ionizing radiation is the oxidation of ferrous ions to ferric ions in solution. Other examples are the change in colour of some dyestuffs. For instance, red perspex is turned black and methylene blue is bleached when irradiated. A number of these chemical changes have been used in dosimetry. They can be used only to measure amounts of radiation rather than the intensity of the radiation.

4. Dosimetric quantities and units

So far we have used a number of loose, everyday words to express an amount of radiation. The only term we have used which has a precise physical meaning is intensity, a term which can be applied to a parallel beam of radiation. The intensity of a beam is the amount of energy crossing unit area, held perpendicular to the direction of propagation, per unit time. This term can be applied to any type of radiation; for instance one can speak of the intensity of a beam of sound or a beam of radio energy. When a beam of ionizing radiation interacts with matter, scattering processes occur and the ionizing particles (charged particles, photons or neutrons) may travel in all directions, even if the incident beam is parallel. A more general term is needed to specify the number of particles in this less restricted situation. We speak of the fluence of particles (Φ) which is the quantity $\delta N/\delta a$ where δN is the number of particles which enter a sphere of cross-sectional area δa. Since we are considering the particles entering through the surface of a sphere the fluence is independent of the direction in which the individual particles are travelling. The rate at which the particles enter the sphere is given by the fluence rate which is equal to $d\Phi/dt$.

Instead of talking about the number of particles entering a small sphere we may be more concerned with the energy carried by them. This is measured by the energy fluence (Ψ) which is equal to $\delta E_{fl}/\delta a$ where δE_{fl} is the total energy, exclusive of rest energy, of all the particles entering a sphere of cross-sectional area δa, i.e., it is the sum of the kinetic energies of charged particles and neutrons and the energy of photons entering the small sphere. The rate at which energy enters the sphere is measured by the energy fluence rate (ψ) where $\psi = d\Psi/dt$. The units of energy fluence rate are the same as those of intensity (watts per square metre) but in this case we are no longer restricted to unidirectional propagation.

These quantities are useful in describing a radiation field, that is, a region which is irradiated with ionizing radiation, irrespective of the direction of motion of the radiation. They are helpful in specifying the number of particles or the energy carried by them. However, although they are fundamental quantities, they are difficult to measure and often do not correlate directly with the effects produced by the radiation. In most instances, especially in biological work, we have no intrinsic interest in either the number of ionizing particles or the energy carried by them. What we are concerned with is some convenient effect of the radiation which can be used as a parameter to correlate with the biological effect produced by the radiation. Experience has shown that most biological effects of ionizing radiations are related to the energy deposited by the radiation per unit mass of the irradiated material.

Referring back to fig. 31 we see that the energy deposited by the radiation is transferred to the medium by charged particles, even if the radiation is not directly ionizing. In the case of photons the energy is deposited by secondary electrons; neutrons deposit their energy by producing recoil nuclei. If a particular ionizing particle passes through the medium without interacting with it, no energy is deposited. For a given fluence, the energy deposited per unit mass of the irradiated material, or absorbed dose as it is called, depends on the nature of the ionizing radiation, its energy, the atomic number of the irradiated material and, to some extent, its density. The energy is deposited by ionization and excitation produced by charged particles and this energy may then produce other effects, such as biological effects, in the medium. We use the absorbed dose as a measure of the other effects produced by the radiation.

Fig. 34 shows an extended medium irradiated with ionizing radiation. This radiation produces charged particles in the medium and these charged particles may travel in any direction, depositing their energy as they pass through the matter. Let us consider a small volume element of the matter of mass δm, which is traversed by some charged particles. These charged particles deposit an amount of energy δE in the small element. The absorbed dose at the element is defined by the ratio $\delta E/\delta m$. The unit of absorbed dose (usually abbreviated to dose) is the gray (Gy) where

$$1 \text{ Gy} = 1 \text{ J kg}^{-1}$$

Fig. 34

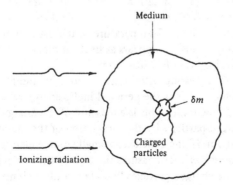

Medium

δm

Charged particles

Ionizing radiation

An older unit of dose, the rad, will be seen in the literature. It was defined in c.g.s. units by 1 rad $= 100$ erg g^{-1}. From these definitions it can be seen that 1 Gy $= 100$ rad.

The following features of the gray should be borne in mind:

(1) It is not a unit of radiation but a unit of the result of the irradiation of matter. It does not measure the primary radiation but the effect this radiation has in depositing energy in matter.

(2) The gray is independent of the material irradiated since it is defined as energy deposited per unit mass. If we take small samples of different materials such as, say, air and lead, and irradiate them independently of each other so that energy is deposited uniformly throughout each of the samples, then the dose to each is the ratio of the energy deposited (in joules) to the mass of material (in kilograms). If we choose the durations of the irradiations to make this ratio the same in the two cases then each of the samples will receive the same number of grays. The fluence of primary radiation may be quite different in the two irradiations. For instance if the radiation used in both cases is low energy X-rays, the air sample will require a much greater fluence than the lead, owing to the greater photoelectric effect in lead, but, nevertheless, both samples will receive the same dose.

(3) The gray is independent of the nature of the primary ionizing radiation.

Although dose is of great importance, especially in biological work, it has the drawback that it is often a difficult quantity to measure directly. To measure the dose at a point in a medium we have to take a small mass of the medium at the point of interest and isolate it from the rest of the medium (without in any way disturbing the radiation field) and measure the energy deposited in this isolated element. In principle this can be done by measuring the change of temperature of the mass, assuming that all the energy deposited appears as heat. In practice it may be difficult to realize this ideal situation.

When dealing with indirectly ionizing radiation a useful radiation quantity is the kerma (kinetic energy released per unit mass in the medium). This is a measure of the energy imparted to charged particles by the interaction of the radiation with the medium. If one considers a small volume element of the medium of mass δm and measures the sum of the initial kinetic energies of all the charged particles liberated in this volume element by indirectly ionizing radiation (δE_{tr}), then the kerma is the ratio δE_{tr} divided by δm. Kerma is measured in the same units as the gray, i.e. joules per kilogram.

The reason for using the quantity kerma is because the interaction of indirectly ionizing radiation with matter is a two-stage process: the radiation first interacts with the matter to produce charged particles and these charged particles then interact with the matter to deposit their energy in it. The former stage is measured by the kerma and the latter by the dose. It may seem at first sight that kerma and dose are equal, but this may not be so. If the primary radiation is, say, photons, these interact with the medium to produce secondary electrons. To measure the kerma we need to measure the sum of the initial kinetic energies of the secondary electrons liberated in a small element of the medium. The secondary electrons may produce some bremsstrahlung and the energy of the bremsstrahlung photons may not be absorbed in the element and thus does not contribute to the dose: but their energy is included in the kerma. Similarly, if the primary photons were of high energy the secondary electrons would have large ranges and would dissipate much of their energy outside the small element in which the kerma was being measured. This energy which is carried away by the secondary electrons does not contribute to the dose at the element. The energy lost from the element may be compensated by secondary electrons entering the element from its surroundings, but this depends on the geometry of the irradiation and the energy of the radiation.

If the primary radiation consists of photons only, we can define another radiation quantity: the exposure. This is defined by the quotient δQ by δm where δQ is the absolute value of the total charge on the ions of one sign produced in the air when all the electrons (electrons and positrons) liberated by photons in a volume element of air having mass δm are completely stopped in air.

$$\text{Exposure} = \frac{\delta Q}{\delta m}$$

The unit of exposure has no name; it is measured in coulombs per kilogram of air.

To interpret the definition of exposure one considers a small volume element of air of mass δm. The primary photons will, when they interact with the air in this volume, produce secondary electrons. These secondary electrons are produced by the photo-

electric process, Compton process, or pair production; they are
energetic particles and may have large ranges. As they pass through
the air they ionize it. From the definition of exposure, all the secondary electrons produced in the volume element must produce
all of their ionization in air. The ions they produce must be pre-
vented from recombining and the total charge carried by the ions
of one sign measured. If the ratio of this charge to the mass of air
in the volume element is 1 C kg^{-1} we have unit exposure.

For historical reasons, and perhaps as a matter of convenience,
a special unit of exposure has been defined. This is the roentgen
(R). It is defined by

$$1 \text{ R} = 2.58 \times 10^{-4} \text{ C kg}^{-1}$$

This is not a true SI unit although it is defined in SI base units. It
is likely to become obsolete in the not too distant future. The
figure 2.58×10^{-4} C kg^{-1} in the definition of the roentgen may
seem very peculiar. It originates from an earlier definition in
terms of the electrostatic unit of charge (3.33×10^{-10} C) and the
mass of 1 cm^3 of air at STP (0.00129 g). Effectively the roentgen
was defined as 1 e.s.u. of charge per cubic centimetre of air. It
will be seen that the old definition amounts to 2.58×10^{-4} C kg^{-1}.
Thus the roentgen defined in SI base units is of the same magnitude as the roentgen in c.g.s. units.

It may seem rather unfortunate that the defining body chose to
redefine the roentgen in SI base units. There was no necessity for
this step since there is no real difficulty in working in a unit of
exposure of 1 C kg^{-1}. The only justification seems to be that there
was already a roentgen (defined in c.g.s. units) and people were
familiar with this unit. Using 1 C kg^{-1} would have involved using
a unit some 3876 times larger than the existing roentgen and all
exposures measured in coulombs per kilogram would have num-
erical values correspondingly smaller.

The old c.g.s. definition of the roentgen explicitly stated that
it was a quantity of X-rays or γ-rays. The new definition no
longer says this. It defines exposure and the roentgen in a similar
way to dose and the gray, but whereas in the definition of dose the
effect produced by the ionizing radiation is the amount of energy
imparted to a small mass and the nature of both the ionizing radiation and the medium are left unrestricted, in the definition of
exposure the effect is the ionization produced by secondary electrons originating in a small mass and the radiation is explicitly
defined (photons) as is the medium (air). So, as with dose,

exposure is a result of the radiation, not a measure of the radiation itself. It may, in fact, be easier to think of exposure as a quantity of X-rays or γ-rays, although this is not strictly true.

The exposure at a point in a medium other than air can also be measured. If one considers a small volume of air in the medium at the point of interest and measures all of the ionization due to secondary electrons originating in that volume, the ratio of the charge carried by ions of one sign to the mass of air in the volume gives the exposure at the point, and this ratio divided by 2.58×10^{-4} gives the exposure in roentgens. It must be stressed, though, that all the ionization from secondary electrons originating in the small volume of air must be measured and all this ionization must be produced in air. Further, no ionization from secondary electrons originating in the rest of the medium must be measured. Provided these conditions are satisfied, the ratio of the charge liberated to the mass of air in the volume gives the exposure at the point of interest in the medium.

Historically, exposure preceded dose as a radiation quantity. The roentgen was originally defined at a time when our understanding of the interaction of radiation with matter was rather rudimentary. The definition was compounded before the discovery of either the neutron or the positron, at a time when there was insufficient evidence to show that biological effects are related to absorbed energy. We now know that it is not the quantity of radiation itself which is important but the energy it deposits per unit mass. We no longer define the roentgen as a quantity of radiation, even if this concept is easier to grasp, but as an effect of photons in matter. The reason for retaining exposure as a radiation quantity is that in practice it is comparatively easy to measure ionization in air compared with most of the other physical effects of radiation, and having measured exposure in a medium it is not too difficult to convert the measurement to absorbed dose in the medium.

The question arises as to why we measure ionization in air rather than any other gas. The answer to this question is two-fold. First, air is a readily available material and its composition is approximately constant all over the surface of the earth, provided that the air is dry. The second reason is more fundamental than this practical consideration. In most biological and medical work using X-rays we irradiate soft tissue such as muscle. The quantity we want to measure is the dose delivered to the tissue by the photons. Since we often cannot measure this quantity directly,

we need some indicator the reading of which is proportional to
the dose delivered for all photon energies. Suppose we have a
quantity of soft tissue (fig. 35) with a small gas-filled cavity in it
containing a mass, δm, of gas. Suppose that the whole mass of
tissue and gas is irradiated uniformly with X-rays. The photons
need not necessarily all come from the same direction, nor need
the individual photons all have the same energy; the only requirement is that the fluence of photons is the same in the gas cavity
as in the surrounding tissue and the energy spectrum of the
photons is the same in both cases. Energy is deposited in both the
tissue and gas by secondary electrons produced by the photoelectric process, Compton process and pair production. We have seen
(pp. 28–39) that these interactions depend on both the atomic
number of the medium and the energy of the photons, but, if
the atomic number of the gas is the same as tissue, the number of
secondary electrons produced per unit mass of the gas is the same
as the number produced per unit mass of tissue and the energy
distribution of the secondary electrons is the same in both cases.
Neglecting the small correction originating from the density
effect, the amount of energy deposited by the secondary electrons per unit mass of the gas is equal to the energy deposited per
unit mass of tissue, and the dose in the two media is the same.
This equality holds whatever the average energy of the photons.
The effective atomic number of soft tissue is 7.4 and that of air is
7.6. Although these two values are not identical they are close
enough for most practical purposes. If air is chosen as the material
to fill the cavity, although the dose to the air will not be identical
to that of the tissue it will closely parallel it over a wide range of

Fig. 35

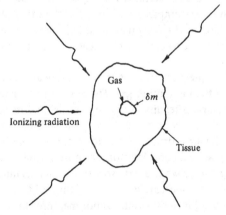

Ionizing radiation

Gas

δm

Tissue

photon energies. Since the average amount of energy required to produce an ion pair in air is independent of the photon energy, the ionization per unit mass of air closely parallels the dose delivered to soft tissue over a wide range of photon energies. In fact the divergence from proportionality is of the order of only ten per cent in the three decades of photon energy from 10 keV to 10 MeV used in most biological and medical work. If the effective atomic number of air were the same as soft tissue, the ionization per unit mass of air would be directly proportional to the dose delivered to the tissue at all photon energies.

The parallelism between ionization in air and tissue holds only if the two effective atomic numbers are about the same. Most soft tissues have approximately the same composition, but bone has a much higher effective atomic number (about 13) and in this case the dose to bone does not parallel ionization in air. At low energies there is a much higher photoelectric absorption in bone ($\tau/\rho \propto Z^3$) and therefore the dose to bone is higher than the dose to air at low energies.

It must be stressed that exposure is a term that can be used only if the beam of radiation consists of photons. The relationship between exposure and dose may be easier to understand if one considers an analogy which, in its original form, was attributed to L.H. Gray. Imagine a lecturer talking to his class. As he burbles on his words spread through the lecture theatre and represent the fluence of photons. Most of his words pass through the students' heads without having any noticeable effect. A few of the words stick on their passage between the ears. These words represent the exposure. The words which stick stimulate the students to think for themselves and these thoughts represent the dose. As with most analogies one must not examine it too closely. When photons interact with matter the dose increases with the density of the medium, but every teacher knows that the converse is true about students' heads.

The relationship between exposure and the gray in air

If one takes a mass m of air and irradiates it with photons to give it unit exposure uniformly throughout its volume, from the definition of unit exposure the total charge on ions of one sign produced in each kilogram of the air is 1 coulomb (C). The charge on the ions of one sign in the mass m is therefore m C. The charge on each ion, either positive or negative, is equal to the charge on the electron (1.6×10^{-19} C) and so the number of ion pairs produced in the mass by unit exposure is equal to

$$\frac{m}{1.6 \times 10^{-19}}$$

We have seen that $\bar{W}$, the average energy required to produce one ion pair, is independent of photon energy. $\bar{W}$ is normally measured in electron volts and so the amount of energy deposited in the mass m is equal to

$$\frac{m \times \bar{W}}{1.6 \times 10^{-19}} \text{ eV}$$

But 1 eV is equal to 1.6×10^{-19} joules (J) and so the energy deposited in the mass m is equal to

$$\frac{m \times \bar{W} \times 1.6 \times 10^{-19}}{1.6 \times 10^{-19}} = m \times \bar{W} \text{ J}$$

The energy deposited per unit mass of air is $\bar{W}$ J and therefore, since 1 Gy = 1 J kg^{-1}, the dose to the air is equal to $\bar{W}$ Gy. The currently accepted value of $\bar{W}$ for air is 33.7 eV per ion pair and so unit exposure is equivalent to a dose of 33.7 Gy in air and is independent of the photon energy. Since the roentgen is about 3876 times smaller than unit exposure, an exposure of 1 R in air is equivalent to a dose of about 8.7×10^{-3} Gy.

Relationship between exposure and the gray for media other than air

Suppose we have (fig. 36) two masses, m_1 of air and m_2 of any other medium, and they are both irradiated with the same fluence of monoenergetic photons. For simplicity, suppose that the beam of photons is parallel. The probability of photons interacting with atoms in the air mass is proportional to the number of atoms in it, which is proportional to its mass. Similarly, the probability is proportional to the photon fluence Φ. Energy is deposited in the air

Fig. 36

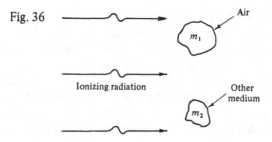

Ionizing radiation

mass by secondary electrons. The probability of deposition is proportional to the mass absorption coefficient $(\mu_{en}/\rho)_{air}$. We use the absorption coefficient, not the attenuation coefficient, because we are concerned with the energy deposited by the photons, not the removal of photons from the beam. Thus, we can write

$$E_{air} = k\Phi(\mu_{en}/\rho)_{air}\, m_1$$

where E_{air} is the energy deposited in the air and k is a constant. Similarly for the medium

$$E_{med} = k\Phi(\mu_{en}/\rho)_{med}\, m_2$$

Thus

$$\frac{E_{med}}{E_{air}} = \frac{(\mu_{en}/\rho)_{med}\, m_2}{(\mu_{en}/\rho)_{air}\, m_1}$$

But E_{air}/m_1 = dose to the air and E_{med}/m_2 = dose to the medium, therefore

$$\frac{Dose_{med}}{Dose_{air}} = \frac{(\mu_{en}/\rho)_{med}}{(\mu_{en}/\rho)_{air}}$$

But we have seen that $dose_{air} = 33.7 \times X$, where X is the exposure in coulombs per kilogram. Therefore we have

$$Dose_{med} = 33.7\frac{(\mu_{en}/\rho)_{med}}{(\mu_{en}/\rho)_{air}} \times X$$

We can write this expression as

$$Dose_{med} = f \times X$$

where

$$f = 33.7\,\frac{(\mu_{en}/\rho)_{med}}{(\mu_{en}/\rho)_{air}}.$$

The term f is called the f-factor of the medium and gives the conversion from exposure in coulombs per kilogram to dose in grays. Thus if we measure the exposure in the medium by ionization produced in air we can calculate the dose to the medium by multiplying the exposure by the f-factor of the medium. If the exposure X is measured in roentgens the f-factor is given by

$$f = 8.7 \times 10^{-3}\,\frac{(\mu_{en}/\rho)_{med}}{(\mu_{en}/\rho)_{air}}$$

The derivation we have used is for a parallel beam, but the

same argument holds if the fluence is of photons travelling in all directions, since the fluence can be thought of as the resultant of a large number of separate parallel beams, each beam having a different direction, and we can use the same absorption coefficient for each of these beams.

Values of the f-factor are plotted in fig. 37 for water, muscle and bone, for exposures measured in both coulombs per kilogram and roentgens. A line is also drawn for air but, as we have seen, this line occurs at a value of 33.7 Gy C^{-1} kg or at 8.7×10^{-3} Gy R^{-1}, independent of the photon energy. The value of the f-factor for the other media depends on the ratio of $(\mu_{en}/\rho)_{med}$ to $(\mu_{en}/\rho)_{air}$ at different photon energies. At energies where the Compton process is the main interaction, bone, muscle, water and air have approximately the same f-factor since their number of electrons per unit mass is roughly the same. Bone, muscle and water have slightly greater f-factors than air in this region because they all contain a certain amount of hydrogen, which has approximately twice as many electrons per unit mass as other elements and gives a correspondingly greater Compton interaction. The graphs illustrate the reason for using air as a dosimetric material. The curves for muscle (a typical soft tissue) and air are approximately parallel over a wide range of photon energies. Bone, with a higher atomic number ($Z \sim 13$), behaves differently. At low energies photons have a much higher photoelectric interaction with bone and so the dose per unit exposure is of the order of four times greater for bone than air or soft tissue. At higher energies, where the photoelectric process is less important ($\tau/\rho \propto \lambda^3$) and most of the interaction is by the Compton process, the dose per unit exposure for bone is about the same as for air and soft tissue. This is the rationale for using high energy photons in situations where bone and soft tissue are irradiated simultaneously. Both the bone and the soft tissue receive approximately the same dose for a given photon fluence. If low energy photons were used the bone would receive four times the dose delivered to the soft tissue.

The graphs also demonstrate why water is frequently used as a material in which to make experimental measurements of dose distributions. As far as its interaction with photons is concerned it behaves nearly the same as soft tissue.

The curves of fig. 37 are drawn for monoenergetic photons. When a heterogeneous beam of X-rays is used the f-factor for converting from exposure to dose is averaged over the range of energies of the photon beam.

Linear energy transfer
Dose is a macroscopic measure of the energy imparted to a medium
by ionizing radiation. Although dose is usually the most important
variable influencing the action of the radiation a number of other
factors may be involved, in particular the microscopic distribution

Fig. 37

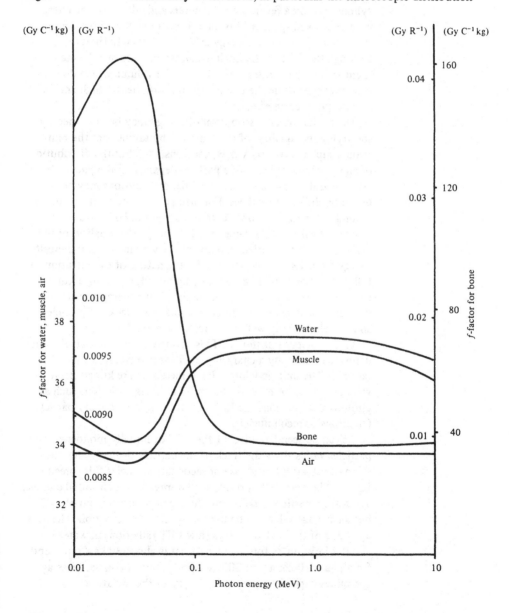

of energy along the paths of the particles. This must be so, for, if
we consider a small volume of matter which is irradiated with,
say, alpha particles, most of the energy lost by each of the individual alpha particles is deposited by ionization and excitation
within a narrow cylinder around its path. The radius of the
cylinder is only a few atomic diameters and, although the energy
is degraded and spreads with time throughout the whole volume,
the initial deposition of energy is highly localized. Therefore,
although the dose to the small irradiated volume may be high,
there are many microscopic regions in the volume which do not
receive energy while the quanta are at a sufficiently high energy
level to produce an effect.

The initial spatial distribution of energy may be described by
specifying the 'quality' of the radiation by saying that the radiation is alpha particles, X-rays, neutrons, etc., but the distribution
of energy along the path of a particle depends on the particle's
velocity and charge, and similar spatial distributions may be produced by different particles. For instance the energy distribution
around the path of a slow electron may be similar to that of a
proton travelling at the same velocity. Hence the 'quality' of the
radiation is best specified in terms of the way in which it deposits
energy along its path rather than by the nature of the radiation. A
full description would be rather complicated, requiring a knowledge of every collision along the path. Linear energy transfer is
used as a single parameter to characterize the tracks of particles
and correlates fairly well with biological effectiveness.

Linear energy transfer (LET) is defined as the amount of energy
deposited locally by a charged particle as it traverses a small distance δl. The units in which LET is measured are kiloelectron
volts per micrometre. With indirectly ionizing radiations such as
photons and neutrons the LET is that of their secondary particles
(electrons or recoil nuclei).

As can be seen from fig. 11 the LET of initially monoenergetic
particles varies along the track of the particle owing to the variation of velocity. In the case of secondary particles this spread of
LET will be emphasized owing to the spread of their initial energies.
Thus, for a particular radiation, there will be a spectrum of LET,
but an average value can be used to specify the radiation. The average value of the LET of X-rays (low LET radiation) in water is
about 7 keV μm^{-1}, for fast neutrons it is about 30 keV μm^{-1} and
for alpha particles about 200 keV μm^{-1}, but of course, these average values depend on the actual energy of the radiation.

5. The measurement of exposure

In order to measure an exposure we need to take a small mass of air, δm (fig. 38) and allow all the secondary electrons produced in this mass by photons to come to rest in air. We must then measure the total charge on ions of one sign produced by these secondary electrons in air. The ratio of this charge to δm is the exposure. If we divide this ratio by 2.58×10^{-4} we will have determined the exposure in roentgens. It will be seen from fig. 38 that many of the secondary electrons originating inside δm produce ionization outside δm. We must measure all of the ionization produced by secondary electrons which originate inside δm, i.e. the sum of the ionization they produce inside and outside δm, without measuring any ionization produced by secondary electrons originating outside δm.

The instrument used to make these measurements is the standard free air ionization chamber (fig. 39). This is an instrument which is used to make absolute determinations of exposure and is used to calibrate other, more convenient ionization chambers. In the instrument a beam of X-rays from a source is restricted laterally by a lead diaphragm. The resulting narrow beam is allowed to pass between a pair of parallel metal plates which have air between them. The upper plate is a continuous metal plate. The lower plate is made in three sections with small gaps between them. The two outer sections of the lower plate are connected to earth and the central section is connected to a charge-measuring electrometer (E) the other side of which is earthed. The upper plate is connected to the negative terminal of a battery the positive terminal of which is also earthed. With this arrangement a potential

Fig. 38

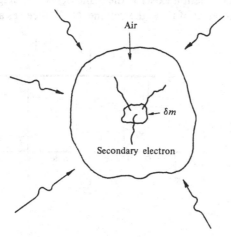

Air

δm

Secondary electron

difference exists between the upper and lower plates equal to the
e.m.f. of the battery. Positive ions produced between the plates
drift along the lines of force to the upper plate and negative ions
drift to the lower plate. The electrometer measures only negative
ions arriving at the central section of the lower plate (the collector electrode). The potentials of all three sections of the lower
plate are the same and with this arrangement the lines of force are
of the form indicated by the broken lines. They are straight,
parallel lines normal to the surfaces of the plates over most of the
volume of the gas between the plates. Towards the edges of the
plates the lines of force bow outwards. The reason for construct-
ing the lower plate in this guarded form is to ensure that all of
the lines of force terminating on the central section DC are
straight lines over the whole of their length. This ensures that the
electrometer measures only ions formed in the region $ABCD$. In
use the electrometer must be operated in such a way that the
potential of DC remains constant and equal to that of its guards,
thus ensuring that the lines of force remain straight. If the
potential of DC is allowed to differ from its guards, the lines of
force at the edges of DC distort and the electrometer no longer
measures all the negative ions produced in $ABCD$.

Let us now consider the ionization produced in the volume
$ABCD$ (fig. 40). Most of this ionization is due to secondary electrons that originate in $PQRS$. But, considering the plane $APSD$,
some secondary electrons originating to the left of this plane produce ionization in the volume $ABCD$ and a few originating in
$PQRS$ travel to the left producing ionization outside $ABCD$. A
similar situation exists at the plane $BQRC$. Averaged over a reasonable interval of time, the volume $ABCD$ receives as much ionization

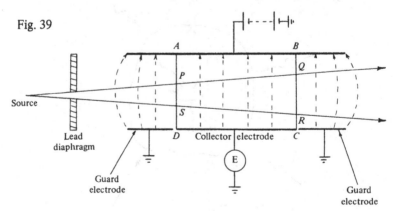

Fig. 39

from secondary electrons originating outside it as it loses due to secondary electrons originating inside *PQRS* but producing some of their ionization outside *ABCD*. Thus, effectively, the volume *ABCD* contains all the ions produced by secondary electrons originating in the volume *PQRS* and the negative ions arrive at the collector *DC*. If the total charge carried by these ions is measured by the electrometer, the value of this charge divided by the mass of air in *PQRS* gives the exposure and this ratio divided by 2.58×10^{-4} gives the exposure in roentgens.

The definition of exposure states that the secondary electrons must all be produced in air. To satisfy this requirement no secondary electrons originating in any material other than air must be allowed to enter the volume *ABCD*. The lead diaphragm used to limit the dimensions of the X-ray beam produces secondary electrons by the attenuation processes. To prevent any of these electrons from entering *ABCD* the distance between the diaphragm and the plane *APSD* is made greater than the maximum range in air of these electrons; thus they are brought to rest in the air to the left of *APSD*. This condition is also necessary to ensure that the plane *APSD* receives its full quota of electrons produced in the air to the left of it to compensate the loss of electrons at plane *BQRC*. The definition also states that all of the ionization produced by the secondary electrons must be measured. This condition implies that the distances *QB* and *RC* must also be greater than the maximum range of the secondary electrons in air so that any secondary electrons travelling towards the metal plates are brought to rest in air before they arrive at the plates. If this condition were not fulfilled some of the secondary electrons would arrive at the plates before they had dissipated all of their energy and had not produced their full amount of ionization in air. A

Fig. 40

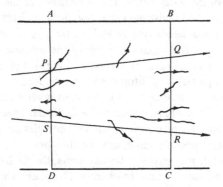

further condition that must be satisfied in order to measure all of
the ionization of the secondary electrons is that no recombination
occurs. The field produced between the plates by the battery
must be sufficiently high to extract all the ions.

It is difficult to determine the mass of air in $PQRS$ directly
since the air in the chamber is open to the atmosphere and consequently its mass fluctuates with atmospheric pressure and temperature. If the volume $PQRS$ is known accurately the mass of air
inside it can be determined by multiplying the volume by the
density of air. Let ρ_0 be the density of air at STP and $\rho_{t,P}$ its density at temperature $t\,^{\circ}C$ and pressure P. From Boyle's and Charles'
laws we know that the mass of a fixed volume of gas is proportional to its pressure and inversely proportional to its absolute
temperature. Therefore

$$\rho_{t,P} = \rho_0 \times \frac{P}{76} \times \frac{273}{(273 + t)}$$

where t is in degrees Celsius and P is in centimetres of mercury.

In practice it is not necessary to measure the volume $PQRS$. If
the source of X-rays is a point source and if attenuation of the
beam in air is negligible, the intensity of the X-ray beam varies
inversely as the square of the distance from the source and the volume of air can be taken as the area of the aperture in the diaphragm
multiplied by the distance between the planes $APSD$ and $BQRC$,
both of which dimensions can be measured accurately. With this
interpretation of the volume, the point at which the exposure is
measured is at the centre of the aperture of the diaphragm.

The free air chamber is a cumbersome device to use. In order
to prevent spurious effects from stray radiation the chamber is
surrounded by a suitable high atomic number shield with apertures for the X-ray beam. The dimensions of the chamber are large
owing to the requirement that the distances between the diaphragm and the air volume and the plates and the air volume are
greater than the maximum range of the secondary electrons produced by the X-rays. An estimate of the size of the chamber for
use at a particular photon energy can be formed by considering
the ranges of monoenergetic electrons in air given in table 2.
Although a beam of photons of a particular energy produces very
few secondary electrons which have energies approaching the
maximum possible value, and the chamber can be made smaller
without introducing substantial errors, the device is nevertheless
large and inconvenient to operate. Chambers which have much
smaller dimensions and which are easier to operate are used for

routine measurements. These chambers, which are made with an air wall, are calibrated against the standard free air ionization chamber at a standardization laboratory.

Air wall ionization chambers

Consider a small sphere of air of mass δm (fig. 41) at the centre of a larger sphere of air, with the whole mass irradiated uniformly with photons. Suppose the radius of the outer sphere is equal to the maximum range, R, in air, of the secondary electrons set in motion by the photons, and the diameter of the inner sphere is small compared with the range of the secondary electrons. Secondary electrons are set in motion throughout the whole of the mass of air. Only a few secondary electrons are set in motion in the small inner sphere because we have specified that it is small and hence it contains relatively few atoms and is traversed by relatively few photons; the probability of the photons interacting within its boundary is low. The secondary electrons originating in the small sphere dissipate only a small fraction of their energy as ionization in the air inside the inner sphere since its diameter is small compared with their range. Most of their ionization is pro-

Table 2. *Ranges of monoenergetic electrons in air*

Electron energy	Range (cm of air at STP)
100 keV	12
500 keV	150
1 MeV	360
5 MeV	2300

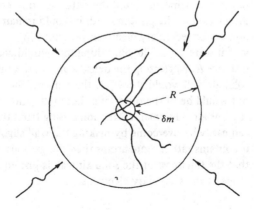

Fig. 41

duced outside in the large outer sphere. The inner volume is traversed by many electrons which originate in the large outer mass
of air. Each of these electrons produces only a small amount of
its ionization in the inner air volume. Averaged over a reasonable
interval of time, the amount of ionization produced in the small
inner sphere by electrons which originate outside it is just equal
to the amount of ionization produced outside it by electrons that
originate inside it. Therefore the total ionization produced inside
the inner sphere is just equal to the amount of ionization due to
secondary electrons which originate inside it. This equality only
holds if the time interval considered is not too short. In a very
short time interval it will not hold owing to the statistical fluctuations in the production of secondary electrons. A further condition for the equality to hold is that the attenuation of the
photons is negligible in the outer sphere, that is, that the attenuation of the photons can be neglected in a thickness of air equal
to the maximum range of their secondary electrons.

If we could measure the charge carried by the ions of one sign
in the small inner sphere and divide this by the mass of air, δm, in
the sphere, this would give the exposure; dividing this by 2.58 ×
10^{-4} would give the exposure in roentgens. We would have satisfied the requirements of the definition of exposure because all of
the ionization produced in the inner sphere is due to secondary
electrons which are produced in air (the thickness of air outside
the inner sphere is equal to the maximum range of the secondary
electrons and so only electrons produced in air can enter the inner
volume) and we would have, in effect, measured the ionization
produced in air by the secondary electrons originating in δm.

The situation would not change if we condensed the air in the
outer sphere into solid air. The number of atoms in it would
remain the same, as would their atomic numbers, and hence the
interaction of the photons with it would remain constant and the
number of secondary electrons produced in it would be the same
as if it were a gas. The only thing that would change would be the
distance R. Neglecting the density effect, the thickness of the
solid air wall would still equal the range of the secondary electrons,
but would be of the order of a thousand times smaller than in
gaseous air. The small correction arising from the density effect
can easily be overcome by making the wall slightly thicker so that
it contains rather more atoms than the gaseous air envelope, so
that the thickness of the solid air wall is just equal to the maximum
range of the secondary electrons.

This hypothetical situation could not be used in a practical ionization chamber where we need the wall to be made of a material rather less evanescent than solid air and where we also need conducting electrodes to collect the ionization. However, if we used a solid material for the wall which interacted with X-rays in exactly the same way as the solid air, which produced exactly the same number of secondary electrons, with exactly the same energy spectrum, for a given photon fluence, then our chamber would satisfy the requirements of the definition of exposure. Such a material is called an air equivalent material and a chamber con-structed of such a material is called an air wall chamber. In order for a material to be air equivalent it must produce the same inter-action with X-rays at all photon energies as air does. We have seen (pp. 28–39) that the three interaction processes depend on the atomic number of the absorber; thus air equivalent materials must have the same effective atomic number as air (7.6).

In order that our chamber may satisfy the requirements of the definition of exposure it is necessary for the inner air volume to receive as much ionization from the outer wall as it loses to it. In effect this means that as many secondary electrons are brought to rest in the small inner volume as are set in motion in it. This con-dition is called electronic equilibrium. Electronic equilibrium pre-vails if the volume of air has dimensions small compared with the range of the secondary electrons and is surrounded by a volume of air of thickness equal to the maximum range of the secondary electrons, and the attenuation of the photons is negligible in a thickness of air equal to the maximum range of their secondary electrons. An air wall ionization chamber can be used to measure exposure only if electronic equilibrium prevails.

The practical air wall chamber
The construction of a practical air wall chamber is illustrated in fig. 42. The outer air wall acts as one electrode and a second elec-

Fig. 42

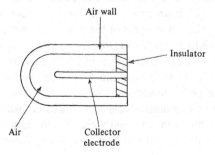

Air wall

Insulator

Air

Collector
electrode

trode along the centre of the chamber acts as the collector. The electrodes are insulated from each other with an insulator of amber or one of the modern plastics. These chambers are often referred to as thimble chambers because of their shape. Various 'magic mixtures' have been used for the construction of the outer wall. The composition of these mixtures is devised on an empirical basis to produce the same interaction as air with photons of all energies. Such a mixture might be made of bakelite loaded with carbon (to make it conducting) with a small amount of higher atomic number material added to increase the effective atomic number to 7.6. The collector electrode in such a chamber is made of the same material as the outer wall. The advantage of using bakelite in the composition is that the electrodes can be moulded to their final shape.

Some chambers have an outer wall made of a plastic, such as bakelite or nylon, and this is rendered conducting by coating its inner surface with graphite. The atomic number of such a wall is of the order of 6 and it produces rather fewer secondary electrons than is required. To compensate for this the inner electrode is made of aluminium ($Z = 13$) which produces an excess of secondary electrons, and the amount of aluminium is adjusted to make the effective atomic number of the chamber as a whole equal to that of air. This adjustment is done empirically by comparing the response of the chamber with that of a standard chamber using X-rays of different energies. If the response of the chamber is too low at low energies the amount of high atomic number material is increased. If the response is too high the amount of high atomic number material is reduced by trimming the central electrode.

Particular care must be taken over the atomic number of the material at the inner surface of the air wall. Small amounts of high atomic number material here have a marked effect on the behaviour of the chamber because this region produces a disproportionately large number of the secondary electrons which traverse the air volume. This is because only high energy secondary electrons produced in the outer layers of the wall can penetrate to the air volume since low energy electrons are absorbed in the wall itself, whereas virtually all of the secondary electrons produced in the layers adjacent to the air volume may traverse it. Small amounts of high atomic number material, present as impurities in the graphite or as mould release agents used in manufacturing the wall, produce a much larger yield of secondary electrons by photoelectric absorption than is required. This is particularly so if the chamber is used to measure exposure due to low energy photons.

A modern development of the graphite-coated plastic wall is to make the whole of the wall from pure graphite by machining it from solid graphite. This construction avoids errors due to impurities on the inner surface of the wall and also prevents troubles that may arise from the graphite coating on a plastic wall not being uniform or becoming detached. The central electrode is of pure aluminium and the adjustment for air equivalence is made in the same way as with the plastic chambers. A further advantage of a graphite chamber is that graphite has greater long term dimensional stability than most plastics and so the volume of the air space, and hence the sensitivity of the chamber, remains more constant with age. Short term fluctuations in the volume of the chamber caused by temperature changes are also very much smaller since graphite has a much smaller coefficient of expansion than plastics. The only disadvantage of a graphite wall is that it is considerably less robust than a plastic wall of the same thickness.

The volume chosen for the air cavity in an air wall chamber depends on the use to which the chamber is to be put. The chamber is connected to some measuring device which measures either the charge liberated in the chamber or the rate at which charge is liberated. For a given sensitivity of the measuring device, the overall sensitivity of the system depends on the volume of the chamber, since a given exposure liberates a charge which is proportional to the mass of air in the chamber. Thus the sensitivity is directly proportional to the air volume. For high sensitivity a large volume is used, but this reduces the spatial resolution of the system since the chamber no longer measures exposure at a small region but gives a value of the average exposure over its entire volume. Commercially manufactured chambers are usually a compromise between high sensitivity and high spatial resolution. They have volumes which range from about 0.1 cm^3 to about 1000 cm^3.

The wall thickness

The number of secondary electrons crossing the air volume in a chamber depends on the thickness of the wall. The major part of the ionization in the air is due to secondary electrons which come from the wall. The ideal wall thickness is such that it just equals the maximum range of the secondary electrons produced by the photons. If the wall is too thin the response of the chamber is too low owing to an insufficiency of electrons produced by the wall.

If the wall is too thick the response is also reduced because of the attenuation of photons in the wall. The situation is illustrated by curve A of fig. 43. This curve is drawn for photons from an X-ray set operating at 200 kVp. The variation of wall thickness is achieved by making a chamber with a very thin wall and then fitting caps of air equivalent material over the chamber. The thickness of wall required for radiation of this energy is taken as the thickness at which the maximum occurs in the curve. For 200 kVp radiation this is of the order of 0.1 mm. If the chamber is irradiated with 15 MV radiation curve B of fig. 43 is produced. Since the secondary electrons have much greater ranges at this energy the wall has to be much thicker, of the order of 3 cm.

It is evident that a different wall thickness is required for measuring exposure from photons of different energies. In practice the manufacturer produces a chamber with a wall of the order of 0.3 mm thick, which is near the ideal for radiation from a 200 kVp source but which is too thick for lower energy radiations. The chamber is calibrated against a standard chamber at different energies and the calibration factor includes the correction for attenuation in the wall. When used to measure exposure with radiation above 200 kVp the wall of the chamber is too thin and electronic equilibrium no longer exists. To rectify this situation a suitable cap of air equivalent material is put over the chamber to increase its wall thickness and give the maximum response. These caps are called 'build-up caps' and are frequently made of perspex. A range of build-up caps is required if the chamber is to be used for different energies above 200 kVp.

Calibration of an air wall chamber
An air wall chamber is not an absolute device and is calibrated

Fig. 43

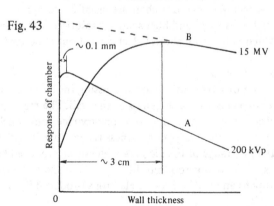

with a standard free air chamber. It is possible to make approximate calculations of either exposure or exposure rate from the charge liberated in the chamber or the ionization current, but these calculations can be only approximate because too many of the variables are not known sufficiently accurately. Although the charge liberated or the ionization current can be measured accurately and attenuation of photons in the wall can be allowed for by extrapolating the curves of fig. 43 back to zero thickness, as is shown by the broken line on curve B, it is difficult to measure the air volume precisely and the air equivalent material is never exactly air equivalent at all photon energies.

In the calibration process a beam of X-rays is allowed to enter the standard free air chamber and the exposure in a given time at the centre of the diaphragm is measured. The standard chamber is then replaced by the air wall chamber. This is placed in the position occupied by the diaphragm of the standard chamber. If the beam of radiation is the same in both cases (same fluence rate and same spectral distribution) the calibration factor is the ratio of the exposure determined with the standard chamber to the reading of the air wall chamber and its measuring device. The process is repeated using beams of radiation of different energy to give a calibration curve for the air wall chamber. A typical calibration curve is shown in fig. 44.

A standard free air chamber can be designed to measure exposure from photons with energies above 10 keV. Below this energy the attenuation of the photons in the air between the diaphragm and the measuring volume is very severe. Above 2 MeV an air wall chamber cannot be used to measure exposure because electronic equilibrium cannot exist, since the attenuation of the

Fig. 44

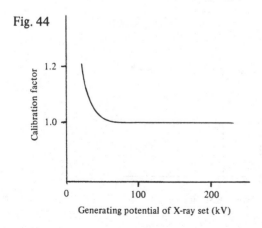

Generating potential of X-ray set (kV)

photons in a thickness of air equal to the range of their secondary electrons can no longer be neglected. Within the range 10 keV to 2 MeV an air wall chamber can be calibrated in roentgens against a standard chamber, but outside this range its reading must be calibrated in terms of another dosimetric quantity such as dose.

Temperature and pressure corrections
If the chamber is sealed the mass of air in it is constant and independent of fluctuations of atmospheric temperature and pressure. Most commercial chambers are not sealed and the mass of air fluctuates with the environmental conditions. During the calibration process the calibration factor of the chamber is corrected to standard conditions. If the chamber is used under different conditions its reading should be corrected to allow for the variation of the mass of gas. If the exposure measured by the chamber after applying the calibration factor is R when the temperature is $t\,°C$ and the pressure P cm of mercury, the corrected reading is

$$\frac{R(t + 273)}{273} \times \frac{76}{P}$$

assuming that the chamber was calibrated at STP.

The collecting voltage and exposure rate
When an ionization chamber is exposed to a constant fluence rate of photons and the collecting voltage applied between the electrodes is varied, the response of the chamber varies with collecting voltage as shown in fig. 45 (curve A). The minimum voltage that must be applied between the electrodes to ensure there is no recom-

Fig. 45

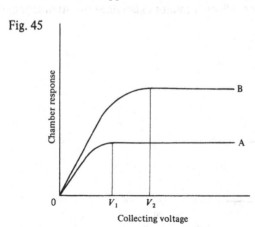

bination is equal to V_1. If the fluence rate is doubled, thus doubling the exposure rate, curve B is produced. Since the average spacing of the ions is less at the higher exposure rate, a greater collecting voltage, in this case equal to V_2, is required to ensure that all the ions are collected. In general the minimum collecting voltage required to prevent recombination increases with the exposure rate. This imposes severe problems when using high exposure rates from pulsed sources. Machines which produce radiation in this way, such as linear accelerators, produce the radiation in short pulses with no radiation between the pulses. The duration of the pulse may be of the order of microseconds and the interval between successive pulses of the order of milliseconds. It is the exposure rate during the pulse which mainly affects recombination and this may be of the order of a thousand times greater than the average exposure rate. Chambers for use with such sources have a small spacing between the electrodes to produce an intense collecting field without necessitating high voltages between the electrodes, but even so it may be difficult to achieve full collection without producing gas multiplication.

Mode of operation of the chamber and its measuring device
There are two ways in which a chamber and its measuring device can be operated. It can be operated in such a way that the charge liberated in the air in a given time is measured. This method gives the exposure. Alternatively the system can be operated in such a way as to measure the rate at which the charge is liberated in the air. This mode of operation gives the exposure rate. In the first method the charge in coulombs on ions of one sign is determined while in the second method the rate of flow of charge in amperes is measured.

Measurement of exposure
Measurement of exposure, by determining the charge liberated, can be achieved in two ways. One way is to treat the chamber as an electrical capacitor of capacitance C (it consists of two electrodes insulated from each other) and charge it to a potential difference V_1 between the electrodes. This will cause a charge Q_1 to flow on to each electrode. The chamber is then removed from the charging device and exposed to radiation. During exposure the ions in the air move to the electrodes and partially neutralize the charge on them. After exposure the charge left on the electrodes is Q_2, where $Q_1 - Q_2$ is equal to the charge carried by ions of

either sign. The charge Q_2 left on the electrodes produces a potential difference V_2 between them. From the definition of capacitance $Q_1 = CV_1$ and $Q_2 = CV_2$. Therefore $Q_1 - Q_2 = C(V_1 - V_2)$. Thus the change in potential difference between the electrodes is directly proportional to the charge carried by the ions, which is directly proportional to the exposure. The device used to measure the initial and final voltages, which must be a high insulation voltmeter, can be calibrated to read exposure directly. This is not a very satisfactory method of measuring exposure since the collecting field decreases during the irradiation and the reduction of the field may allow recombination to occur. The method is used in some chambers used for personnel monitoring, where the exposure rates are expected to be low. Fig. 46 illustrates such a chamber. The instrument has a self-contained electrometer to measure the change in voltage. The lower portion of the instrument is the ionization chamber which has a removable cap for charging. The collector electrode of the chamber is connected to a quartz fibre which deflects under the influence of the potential difference between the collector electrode and the case of the instrument. The fibre is viewed with a microscope which contains a scale calibrated in roentgens. An image of the fibre is formed on the scale, which is so calibrated that when the instrument is fully charged the reading is zero roentgens.

A more satisfactory method of measuring the charge liberated is to use a circuit the principle of which is shown in fig. 47. In

Fig. 46

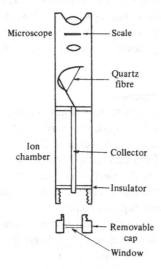

this circuit, charge liberated in the ionization chamber accumu-
lates on the capacitor C and the potential difference developed
across C by this charge is directly proportional to the exposure.
The switch S is included to discharge the capacitor before making
a measurement. The voltmeter used to measure the potential difference across C must have a high input impedance in order that
any current flowing through it is negligible compared with the
current which flows in the ionization chamber during irradiation.
Electronic voltmeters used for this purpose usually have input
impedances of the order of 10^{14} ohm. An advantage of using this
circuit is that the sensitivity of the system, measured by the
change in potential difference across C for a given exposure, is
inversely proportional to C, and by incorporating a range of
capacitors in the instrument its sensitivity can be changed at will.
The two leads WX and YZ are usually in the form of a high
insulation co-axial cable and can be of any convenient length;
thus the measuring unit can be situated at a distance from the
chamber, away from the source of radiation.

Measurement of exposure rate
The ionization current in a chamber is directly proportional to the
exposure rate and the volume of the chamber. An estimate of the
magnitude of the current can be formed by taking a typical
example. Suppose a chamber of volume 1 cm^3 is irradiated with
X-rays and the exposure rate is 10 R per minute. From the
definition of the roentgen this exposure rate causes the liberation
of charge of one sign equal to $10 \times 2.58 \times 10^{-4}$ C in each kilogram of air in the chamber per minute. The density of air is of the
order of 1.29 kg m^{-3} and so the mass of air in the chamber is
equal to 1.29×10^{-6} kg, thus the charge liberated in each minute
is equal to $10 \times 2.58 \times 10^{-4} \times 1.29 \times 10^{-6}$ C. Therefore the
charge liberated per second is

$$\frac{10 \times 2.58 \times 10^{-4} \times 1.29 \times 10^{-6}}{60} C \simeq 5.5 \times 10^{-11} \text{ C}$$

Fig. 47

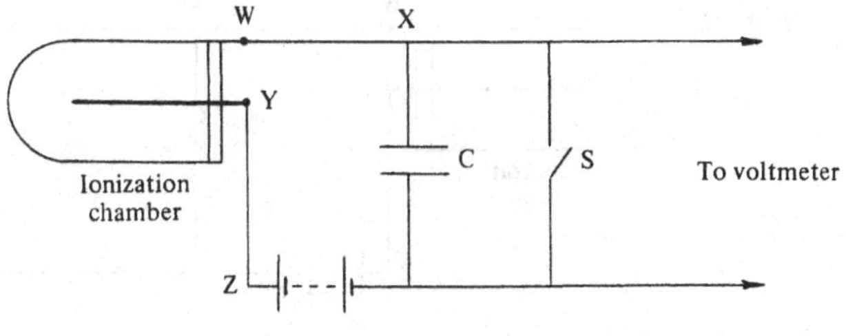

A rate of flow of charge of 1 C per second is equal to a current of 1 ampere (A), therefore the ionization current is of the order of 5.5×10^{-11} A.

The problem of measuring such low currents is overcome by allowing the current to pass through a high value resistor and measuring the potential difference developed across this resistor. The principle of the circuit used is shown in fig. 48; it is similar to that of fig. 47 with the capacitor and shorting switch replaced by the resistor R. If we choose a large value for this resistor the potential difference developed across it by the ionization current has a value which is readily measured. Say we chose R to be 10^{11} ohm, then, in our example, the potential difference across R is of the order of $5.5 \times 10^{-11} \times 10^{11}$ which is equal to 5.5 volts (V). The voltmeter used to measure the potential difference across R must have a high input impedance in order to avoid shunting R. In our example the input impedance would need to be of the order of 10^{13} ohm in order to measure the current, and hence the exposure rate, with 1 per cent accuracy.

The circuit in fig. 48 illustrates the principle of measuring the ionization current and, as with the circuit of fig. 47, the inter-connecting wires WX and YZ can be in the form of a long co-axial cable. If the circuit is used in this form it suffers from the dis-advantage of having a long time constant and the response of the meter indicating the ionization current is very slow. The resistor R is in series with the capacitance of the interconnecting cable and the ion chamber and so the response of the meter is an exponential function of time with a time constant RC where C is the total capacitance in series with R. Taking a typical value of C about 500 picofarads (pF), the time constant with $R = 10^{11}$ ohm is 50 s. It requires a few time constants for the meter to settle down to its steady reading, which, in our example, would be a few minutes. This is obviously undesirable since it would take a long time to make measurements and the instrument could not respond to rapid fluctuations of exposure rate. The voltmeter used to

Fig. 48

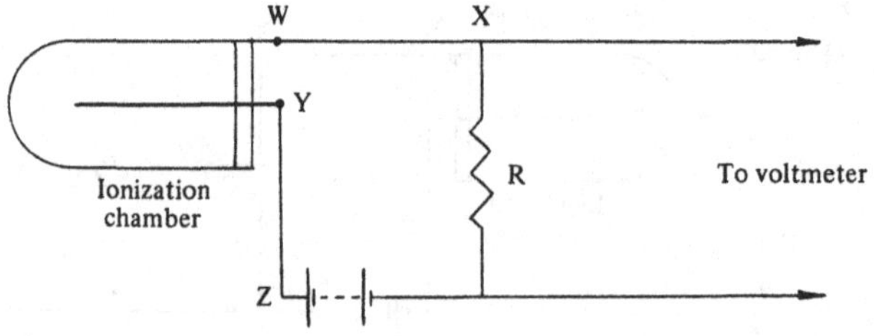

measure the potential difference across R is an electronic device containing an amplifier. To reduce the time constant of the circuit, R is inserted in a negative feedback line in the amplifier. This effectively reduces the time constant to RC/G, where G is the gain of the amplifier. With a typical amplifier gain of the order of 100 the time constant in our example would be reduced to about half a second.

In practice, measurements of both exposure and exposure rate, illustrated in figs. 47 and 48, can be made with the same instrument by incorporating a switch which can select either a suitable resistor or capacitor.

Rough calculations with ionization chambers

As mentioned on p. 75, calculations made with air wall chambers can only be approximations. If one wishes to calculate exposure it is necessary to calculate the charge liberated by the radiation and divide this by the mass of air in the chamber. If this ratio is divided by 2.58×10^{-4} C kg^{-1} the exposure is given in roentgens. Calculation of exposure rate involves calculating the ionization current in coulombs per second (amperes). Dividing this by the mass of air in the chamber gives the exposure rate and, if desired, dividing this value by 2.58×10^{-4} gives the exposure rate in roentgens per second.

As an example, suppose we use an air wall chamber to measure exposure in the method described on p. 77. Suppose the volume of the chamber is 5 cm^3, its electrical capacitance is 10 pF and it is initially charged to a potential difference of 300 V between the electrodes. During exposure the potential difference drops to 200 V. What is the exposure in roentgens if the density of air is 1.29 kg m^{-3}?

First, calculate the charge liberated in the chamber. Since capacitance equals charge divided by potential difference, the initial charge on one electrode of the chamber is equal to $10 \times 10^{-12} \times 300$ C and the final charge is $10 \times 10^{-12} \times 200$ C. Therefore the charge liberated by the radiation is the difference between these two values, which equals 10^{-9} C.

Next, calculate the mass of air in the chamber. The density of air is 1.29 kg m^{-3} and the volume of the chamber is 5 cm^3 = 5×10^{-6} m^3. Therefore the mass of air is $5 \times 10^{-6} \times 1.29$ kg. Therefore the exposure is 10^{-9} C divided by $5 \times 10^{-6} \times 1.29$ kg which equals 1.55×10^{-4} C kg^{-1}. Dividing this by 2.58×10^{-4} C kg^{-1} to give the exposure in roentgens, we have 0.601 R.

6. Methods of measuring dose

Ionization method based on the Bragg–Gray cavity theory

In chapters 4 and 5 we developed a method of determining the dose in a medium by using a calibrated air wall ionization chamber in conjunction with the f-factor of the medium. Although this method can be used in many circumstances, it is restricted since it can only be used for photons in the energy region in which the chamber can be calibrated and measurements can only be made under conditions of electronic equilibrium. The Bragg–Gray theory leads to a method of measuring dose in a medium which, in principle, can be used for any ionizing radiation and is not restricted to situations where electronic equilibrium prevails.

Suppose we have a medium containing a small region of different density or atomic number (fig. 49). This region is referred to as a cavity since in practice it is often gas-filled. Suppose the medium is irradiated with ionizing radiation which could be photons, neutrons or electrons, etc. The medium and cavity are both traversed by charged particles which may be the primary particles themselves or may be secondary particles, such as secondary electrons or recoil nuclei, produced by the interaction of the primary radiation with the medium. Suppose the dimensions of the cavity are so small that the fluence of charged particles in the medium adjacent to the cavity is uniform and the introduction of the cavity into the medium does not affect the fluence of charged particles or their energy spectrum.

Consider one of the charged particles which passes through both the medium and the cavity. The amount of energy it loses per unit path length in the medium is proportional to the stopping power, dE/dx, of the medium and the energy it loses per unit path length in the cavity is proportional to the stopping power of the cavity material. Consider now a fluence, Φ, of charged particles in the medium and suppose that the particles are monoenergetic so that each particle has the same stopping power in the medium.

Fig. 49

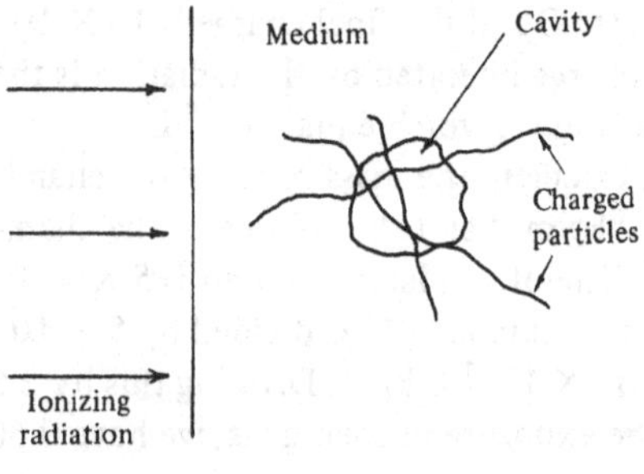

Medium   Cavity

Charged particles

Ionizing radiation

The fluence of particles in the cavity is also Φ since we have specified that the cavity is so small that its introduction does not affect the fluence. The total energy lost by particles per unit volume of the medium is $\Phi(\mathrm{d}E/\mathrm{d}x)_{\mathrm{med}}$ and the energy lost per unit volume of the cavity is $\Phi(\mathrm{d}E/\mathrm{d}x)_{\mathrm{cav}}$. Since the volume occupied by unit mass of a material is inversely proportional to its density, ρ, the energy lost by the particles in unit mass of the medium is equal to $\Phi(\mathrm{d}E/\mathrm{d}x)_{\mathrm{med}}(1/\rho)_{\mathrm{med}}$ and the energy lost by the particles in unit mass of the cavity is equal to $\Phi(\mathrm{d}E/\mathrm{d}x)_{\mathrm{cav}} \times (1/\rho)_{\mathrm{cav}}$.

Assuming that the energy lost by the particles is all transferred to the material of the medium or cavity close to the site where each atomic collision takes place, we can say that the energy lost by the particles in unit mass of material is equal to the dose and so we have the relationship

$$\frac{\mathrm{Dose}_{\mathrm{med}}}{\mathrm{Dose}_{\mathrm{cav}}} = \frac{\Phi(1/\rho \cdot \mathrm{d}E/\mathrm{d}x)_{\mathrm{med}}}{\Phi(1/\rho \cdot \mathrm{d}E/\mathrm{d}x)_{\mathrm{cav}}}$$

$1/\rho.\mathrm{d}E/\mathrm{d}x$ is called the mass stopping power; it is analogous to the mass attenuation coefficient for photons in the sense that it is measured in metres squared per kilogram. So we can say that

$$\frac{\mathrm{Dose}_{\mathrm{med}}}{\mathrm{Dose}_{\mathrm{cav}}} = \frac{S_{\mathrm{med}}}{S_{\mathrm{cav}}}$$

where S_{med} is the mass stopping power of the medium and S_{cav} is the mass stopping power of the cavity.

If the cavity is filled with a gas, the dose to the cavity produces ionization in the gas. Suppose the number of ion pairs produced in unit mass of the gas is I_{gas} and the average energy required to produce one ion pair is $\overline{W}_{\mathrm{gas}}$, then the dose to the gas is equal to $I_{\mathrm{gas}}\overline{W}_{\mathrm{gas}}$ and we have

$$\mathrm{Dose}_{\mathrm{med}} = \frac{S_{\mathrm{med}}}{S_{\mathrm{gas}}} I_{\mathrm{gas}}\overline{W}_{\mathrm{gas}}$$

where S_{gas} is the mass stopping power of the gas. This is the Bragg–Gray relationship and if we measure the ionization in unit mass of the gas we can use it to determine the dose in the medium provided that we know S_{med}, S_{gas} and $\overline{W}_{\mathrm{gas}}$.

In our derivation of the Bragg–Gray relationship we assumed, for simplicity, that all the charged particles traversing the cavity and the medium near the cavity were of the same energy. The same relationship applies if the particles have a spectrum of energies but in this case we use average values of the mass stopping powers in the medium and cavity, averaged over the whole spectrum of particle energies.

In applying the Bragg–Gray relationship to determine dose we construct an ionization chamber to measure the amount of ionization per unit mass of the gas. The chamber must be so constructed that all the ionization produced in the gas is measured, since one has to rely on a measurement of the volume of the cavity of the chamber to give the mass of gas. For this reason it is essential that the chamber is so designed that the field throughout the gas volume is adequate to prevent any recombination and there are no 'dead spaces' where the field is weak and allows ions to recombine. To deduce the dose from the measurement of the ionization we need to know the ratio of the mass stopping powers in the wall of the chamber and the gas. Values of this ratio are most easily deduced if the gas has the same atomic composition as the cavity wall, since in this case the two mass stopping powers differ only by the correction for the density effect. If the walls of the chamber differ from the medium a further complication is introduced since the Bragg–Gray relationship gives the dose to the walls of the chamber. In some situations, such as irradiation with photons, this may not present a problem. In an attempt to reduce uncertainties in the measurements chambers have been constructed with tissue equivalent walls containing tissue equivalent gases.

It is worth looking back at the steps involved in deducing the Bragg–Gray relationship, in particular, the step where we assumed that the energy lost by the charged particle is deposited in the medium close to the site where the particle lost its energy. This assumption is only an approximation since two types of particle collision can lead to energy deposition at a distance. If the charged particle undergoes radiative collision, the energy of the photon is not deposited in the medium close to the site of the interaction and, similarly, in inelastic collisions involving high energy transfer the delta ray carries energy away from the site of the collision. Radiative collisions are allowed for by using values of the stopping power due to inelastic collisions alone, but energy transfer to delta rays presents a greater problem and a number of refinements of the original Bragg–Gray theory have been made in recent years to allow for this effect.

Radiation calorimetry

When ionizing radiations enter matter the energy they deposit appears as thermal energy of the medium and the dose can be determined by measuring the change of temperature produced by this energy. Calorimetric techniques are not confined to ionizing radiation; for instance it is possible to measure the intensity of a microwave beam by absorbing it in water and measuring the temperature change produced by the radiation.

The ion chamber methods of determining dose which we have presented require a knowledge of quantities which are often not known precisely. In the Bragg–Gray method one needs to know the mass stopping powers of the medium and the gas in the cavity and also the value of $\bar{W}$ for the gas. In the calibrated air wall chamber method one needs to know the f-factor of the medium and the calibration factor of the chamber. In both of these ionization methods it is necessary to collect all the ionization produced by the radiation. This imposes a restriction on the use of ionization measurements in situations where the ions are formed very close together in the gas, such as measurements at very high dose rates or with particles which are densely ionizing. In the calorimetric method the temperature rise is independent of the dose rate, depending only on the dose, and the method can, in principle, be used for any ionizing particles.

The temperature rise is often small and this limits the sensitivity of the technique. Consider a mass m kg of matter that has received a uniform dose D Gy. The energy deposited in the mass is mD J. If the specific heat capacity of the matter is c J kg^{-1} K^{-1}, the change in its thermal energy is mct where t is the change of temperature. Since this is equal to the energy deposited by the radiation we have

$$mD = mct \text{ and } t = D/c$$

Thus the temperature change is independent of the mass of matter irradiated. For a large rise in temperature we need c of the material to be small. Taking lead as an example of a material with a low specific heat capacity (~ 130 J kg^{-1} K^{-1}) the temperature rise for a dose of 1 Gy is of the order of 0.008 degrees. With materials of higher specific heat capacity the temperature rise is correspondingly smaller. One of the problems of radiation calorimetry is how to measure such small temperature changes accurately. The most commonly used thermometer is a thermistor used in a similar fashion to a platinum resistance thermometer, in one arm of a Wheatstone bridge. A thermistor is made of metallic oxides and can be formed into a small bead. It is a semiconductor with a large negative temperature coefficient of resistance, of the order of four per cent per degree. Using a thermistor as the thermometer it is possible, with a suitably designed calorimeter, to measure doses of the order 0.5 Gy with moderate accuracy.

The general construction of a radiation calorimeter is illustrated in fig. 50. It consists of a block of calorimetric material surrounded by a jacket designed to minimize heat transfer between the calorimetric material and its surroundings. Embedded in the calorimetric block are one or more thermistors to act as temperature sensors and a small heating coil. In use, radiation is absorbed in the block and produces a temperature change. The amount of energy deposited by the radiation is determined by subsequently dissipating a measured amount of electrical energy in the heating coil to produce the same change of temperature. The advantage of making the measurement of energy in this way is that the measurement does not depend on a knowledge of the thermal capacity of the calorimetric block.

When a calorimeter is used to determine dosimetric quantities it is essential that all the energy deposited by the radiation appears as thermal energy, producing either a change of temperature or a change of physical state of the calorimetric block. The material chosen for the block must be such that no energy is locked up in chemical or physical changes that do not contribute to the change of temperature or state.

The precision of measurement with a calorimeter depends not only on the sensitivity of the detector used to measure the change of temperature or state produced by the radiation but also on the amount of heat transferred between the calorimetric block and

Fig. 50

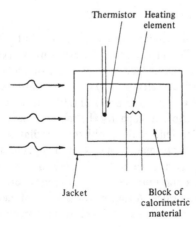

Thermistor   Heating element

Jacket

Block of calorimetric material

its surroundings and the accuracy with which corrections for this heat transfer can be made. Clearly, no heat transfer will occur if the temperature of the jacket is varied during the operating cycle so that it is always the same as the calorimetric block. This is the adiabatic system of calorimetry. The jacket is surrounded by a mantle around which is wrapped a heating element. This heating element is controlled by a servo-mechanism which is operated by the difference of temperature between the calorimetric block and the jacket. Unfortunately the temperature of the jacket tends to oscillate about the temperature of the block and although heat transfer is small it is difficult to calculate accurately. A variation of the adiabatic system is the quasi-adiabatic calorimeter in which the temperature of the jacket is maintained at a small fixed difference from the block. Although heat exchange between the block and its surroundings is larger than in the adiabatic system, it can be allowed for more accurately.

An alternative method of reducing heat transfer is to operate the calorimeter isothermally. In this mode of operation energy deposited by the radiation produces a change of state of the calorimetric material without change of temperature and the energy deposited is determined from the amount of material which changes its state. The principle of operation is similar to the Bunsen ice calorimeter. An inner vessel containing a mixture of ice and water is surrounded by an outer jacket also containing ice and water. On irradiation, some of the ice in the inner vessel melts producing a change of volume without a change in temperature and the energy deposited is determined from this change of volume. Since the inner and outer vessels are at the same temperature the net flow of energy between them is virtually zero. The disadvantage of the ice calorimeter is that it takes a long time for the system to settle down before the small change of volume can be measured accurately. A recent variation of the isothermal calorimeter, using the larger change of volume that occurs between the liquid and gas phases, has been used to measure the stopping powers of charged particles by using their energy to evaporate liquid helium.

A third mode of operation of a calorimeter is the constant-temperature-environment system. In this system the outer layer of the jacket is kept at a constant temperature throughout the operating cycle. The jacket is constructed so as to minimize heat exchange and the correction for heat loss is calculated from the laws of heat flow. This type of calorimeter can be used only in

situations where the rise of temperature of the block occurs
rapidly.

A calorimeter can be used to measure two dosimetric quantities, dose or energy fluence. In measurement of dose the material
used for the absorber is of low atomic number, such as carbon.
The absorber is of small dimensions and the jacket and mantle are
of the same material with only small gaps between the absorber,
jacket and mantle. The gaps are made small to prevent disturbance
of the radiation field. The whole calorimeter is placed in a large
block of the same material. If an identical block is made with a
space for an ionization chamber, the calorimeter and ion chamber
can be irradiated under identical conditions so that their responses
can be compared. This method will probably be used for calibrating ion chambers for use with electron beams and high energy
photons.

Measurements of energy fluence are made by choosing the
material and dimensions of the absorber to completely absorb the
radiation. Thus the temperature rise of the absorber is proportional
to the total amount of energy incident upon it.

Chemical dosimetry
Many chemical systems which respond to ionizing radiation have
been used as dosemeters. It is possible, by choosing suitable systems, to measure doses in the range $0.1-10^8$ Gy. The most frequently used chemical dosemeter (the Fricke dosemeter) is an
aerated dilute solution of ferrous sulphate in sulphuric acid. When
irradiated the ferrous ions are oxidized to ferric ions. In this system the charged particles react initially with water molecules to
produce radicals which then react with oxygen and ferrous sulphate to give ferric sulphate, the concentration of ferric ion
increasing proportionally with dose as long as oxygen remains in
the solution.

The concentration of ferric ion can be determined by direct
titration of the solution or alternatively by measuring the amount
of absorption it produces in a beam of ultraviolet light in a spectrophotometer. Absorption spectroscopy is usually the more convenient method of determining the ferric concentration since it is
a rapid and accurate method and can be applied to low concen-
trations and small volume samples. The absorption of ultraviolet
light in a ferric solution shows a peak at 304 nm, but since the
absorption is temperature dependent the cell containing the ferric
solution should be temperature controlled for precise measurements.

The yield of a radiation induced reaction is specified in terms of its G value. This is the number of molecules produced by 100 eV of absorbed energy. The G value of the Fricke dosemeter is about 15.6, but the precise value depends on the LET of the radiation used. The temperature at which the irradiation is done has little effect on the G value in the temperature range $10\,^{\circ}C$ to $50\,^{\circ}C$, but after the oxygen in the solution has been consumed the G value drops to about 8.

Determinations of the G value have been made by measurement of the energy deposited by the radiation either calorimetrically or by ionization chamber measurements. In the calorimetric method a glass bulb containing water is used as the calorimetric block and the temperature rise in the water under standard radiation conditions is measured. The bulb is then emptied and filled with the Fricke solution and irradiated under identical conditions. Thus the amount of ferric ion produced by a given energy deposition is determined. In the calorimetric determination, with the bulb filled with water, the bulb and its contents are pre-irradiated with a suitably large dose to produce an equilibrium concentration of the radiolytic products in water. This is necessary to ensure that none of the energy is trapped by chemical reactions in the water.

Certain precautions are necessary in the use of the Fricke dosemeter. It is essential to maintain cleanliness, and, in particular, steps must be taken to prevent contamination with organic materials since their presence affects the yield of ferric ions. To this end water used for the solutions and for washing apparatus is triply distilled from an oxidizing solution.

With care the Fricke dosemeter can be used to measure dose with an accuracy of the order of two per cent. The working range of the dosemeter is between 40 and 400 Gy, the lower value being set by the sensitivity of the system used to measure the ferric concentration and the upper limit by the consumption of oxygen in the reaction. Doses lower than 40 Gy can be measured by increasing the sensitivity of the spectrophotometer by increasing the path length of the ultraviolet light in the measuring cell. At low doses the presence of organic impurities becomes more critical and it is preferable to use glass containers rather than plastic irradiation vessels. Doses above 400 Gy can be measured using the 'super' Fricke system which contains a higher concentration of both ferrous sulphate and oxygen, but in this system the G value is increased to 16.1 by the higher oxygen concentration.

Dose rate and LET of the radiation both affect the sensitivity of the Fricke system since at high dose rates or with high LET radiation the radicals formed initially in the water may be produced very close together and consequently radical—radical reactions may compete with the reactions between radicals and the ferrous sulphate, reducing the G value.

Fricke dosimetry is used extensively in radiation chemistry and can be applied to measure the average dose in an irregularly shaped volume. An important application is in calibrating air wall ionization chambers used for making measurements with electron beams, or photons of energy greater than 2 MeV, two fields in which the air wall chamber cannot be calibrated against a standard chamber.

7. Thermoluminescent and photographic dosimetry

Thermoluminescent dosimetry

A thermoluminescent material is one which stores some of the energy dissipated in it by ionizing radiation and releases it as light when heated. The amount of energy trapped and the light emitted depend on the dose received and therefore, by measurement of the light emitted, the material can be used as a dosemeter. Such a system is known as a thermoluminescent dosemeter (TLD).

When a charged particle passes through a thermoluminescent material the interaction of its charge with the atoms of the material causes the ejection of electrons from the atoms (ionization) leaving holes in the atomic structure (i.e. a deficit of electrons). The ejected electrons and holes are free to wander about in the lattice and most of them recombine in a very short interval of time. Some of the electrons or holes may become trapped at imperfections in the lattice structure and remain trapped for long periods of time. In this condition the material has an excess of energy since charge has been separated by the radiation. Raising the temperature of the material may allow the electrons and holes to escape from the traps, and on recombination they give up their surplus energy as light.

The situation may be illustrated by the analogy sketched in fig. 51. In (a) we have a boulder perched on top of a mountain which has a smooth convex top. The boulder is unstable and the principle of minimum energy tells us that it will roll down the mountain to the bottom where its potential energy is least. Now, imagine a mountain with a depression at the top, as shown in fig. 51(b). A boulder in this depression is stable as long as it is not given enough energy to raise it to the rim of the depression. In effect it is trapped in a potential well and is said to be in a metastable state. If, by some means, it is given enough energy to elevate it to the rim of the depression, it will roll down the mountain until

Fig. 51   (a)   (b)

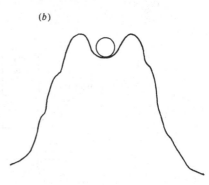

its potential energy is a minimum. The deeper the depression (or the deeper the trap) the greater the energy that must be supplied to the boulder to free it. The condition illustrated in fig. 51(*a*) is analogous to most of the electrons and holes produced by the radiation; they minimize their energy promptly by recombining. The situation of fig. 51(*b*) illustrates an electron or hole trapped by a lattice imperfection. It stays in this state until it is given enough energy by heating to free it.

The traps in a crystal lattice may be due to the presence of impurity atoms or ions (either positive or negative) or they may be due to localized lattice imperfections such as vacancies or dislocations.

Since the majority of the electrons and holes produced by the radiation recombine and only a few are trapped, the efficiency of the system, expressed as the ratio of the energy of the thermoluminescent light to the energy deposited by the ionizing radiation, is low, of the order of one per cent, and it requires a photomultiplier tube to measure the light. The 'read-out' apparatus is shown schematically in fig. 52. The thermoluminescent material is placed in a metal pan which is heated electrically. In order to prevent the photomultiplier tube responding to the thermal radiation from the pan and thermoluminescent material, a filter, which is opaque to infrared radiation but transparent to the thermoluminescent light, is placed between the sample and the photomultiplier tube. The output from the collector of the photomultiplier is taken to an indicator which may be a chart recorder or a digital display. Since the final output of the system depends on the overall gain, which may be rather variable, a weak light source is used as a constant reference. This may take the form of a long-lived β-emitter used in conjunction with a scintillator.

Fig. 52

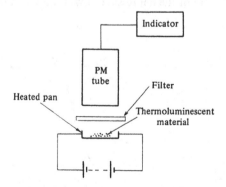

If the photomultiplier output is plotted as a function of the temperature of the irradiated thermoluminescent material the resulting graph is known as a glow curve (fig. 53). The glow curve of a particular material may show a number of peaks; those at low temperature are due to shallow traps which require only a small amount of energy to release the trapped electrons or holes and those at high temperature are due to deep traps. Either the height of the peak in the glow curve or the total amount of light emitted during the heating cycle may be used as an indication of the dose received by the material. The latter is the most common procedure, the heating being arranged so that the pan is taken through a temperature cycle automatically and an integrating circuit is used to sum the output of the photomultiplier tube.

After passing through the temperature cycle required for 'read-out' the thermoluminescent material is ready for re-use, since the traps have been emptied. In practice, if the material is to be re-used, it is usually first taken through an annealing temperature cycle.

Various materials are used as thermoluminescent dosemeters, the principal ones being lithium fluoride, lithium borate activated with a small amount of manganese, calcium fluoride and calcium sulphate. Although the calcium salts give a higher light yield for a given exposure than the two lithium salts, their effective atomic numbers are high (of the order of 16) and consequently their

Fig. 53

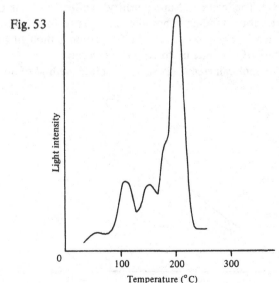

response shows a marked energy dependence when irradiated with photons in the low energy range. Lithium fluoride and borate have effective atomic numbers of 8.2 and 7.4 respectively and their response to photons of different energies is not too different from that of soft tissue. Both lithium fluoride and borate are available as loose powder or as powder embedded in a teflon matrix which is formed into small rods, of the order of 5 mm long and 1 mm diameter, or alternatively as small discs. Lithium fluoride can also be obtained as cleaved crystals. When used in the powder form the material may be encapsulated in a small gelatin capsule similar to those used for pharmaceutical preparations. To read-out the irradiated powder a small amount of it is dispensed into the pan. Since the light output depends on the amount of powder the weight must be accurately controlled. One of the advantages of using the material in the powdered form is that the read-out requires only about 30 mg of material and so a single capsule may be used to give a number of readings.

The variation of the light yield with dose given to the sample is shown in fig. 54 for lithium fluoride. The response is linear up to about 10 Gy but beyond this level the sensitivity increases and the response is 'supralinear'. There is a marked loss of sensitivity with doses above 100 Gy; this is believed to be due to damage in the lithium fluoride produced by the radiation. The useful working range of lithium fluoride is from about 20–30 μGy to about 10^3 Gy. The region of 'supralinearity' is affected by the LET of the radiation, tending to become more nearly linear with increasing LET. The response to low LET radiation is thought to be independent of dose rate up to 10^9 Gy per second.

Thermoluminescence is not an absolute method of dosimetry

Fig. 54

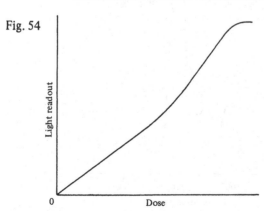

and must be calibrated against some standard dosemeter. The calibration is preferably carried out using the same radiation as it is intended to measure. Since the light yield of a thermoluminescent material depends on imperfections in the crystal lattice, either occurring naturally or produced by artificial doping, the sensitivity of the material tends to vary from batch to batch. The sensitivity may also vary with the previous irradiation history of the material; with, say, lithium fluoride, the sensitivity decreases if the material has previously been given high doses. For this reason it is necessary to calibrate each batch and it is preferable not to mix batches together, especially if they have different irradiation histories.

When the whole of a batch of thermoluminescent material has been used it may be annealed and used again. With the high cost of some materials financial considerations may necessitate re-use. With lithium fluoride powder the annealing cycle is 1 hour at 400 °C followed by 24 hours at 80 °C. When used embedded in teflon, lower temperatures are used to prevent effects in the teflon. The reason for the prolonged annealing at 80 °C is to reduce the effects of shallow traps which show their presence as the low temperature peaks of fig. 53. Since these traps are shallow they may be emptied by thermal agitation at room temperature, causing a fading of the signal. The fading of the low temperature peaks can be speeded up by pre-heating the sample to 100 °C for 5 minutes before read-out. Alternatively the read-out can be delayed for about 24 hours to allow these traps to decay to negligible proportions. The main peaks in the signal, which occur at about 200 °C, also fade with time but this fading is very much slower, of the order of five per cent in 3 months.

Surface effects can also influence thermoluminescent output. These effects may be due to adsorbed gases or to the effects of friction on the surface of the crystals. The light produced by these effects is known as triboluminescence and is suppressed in powder samples by carrying out the heating cycle of the read-out in a stream of nitrogen gas.

The main fields of application of thermoluminescent dosimetry, apart from routine clinical measurements, are in personnel monitoring and in situations where the gradient of a radiation field is steep. In personnel monitoring lithium fluoride has the great advantage that its response does not vary much with the energy of the radiation, much less than that of a photographic emulsion, and its sensitivity is adequate for most protection measurements. In situations where the radiation gradient is steep, i.e. the field is varying rapidly with distance, thermoluminescent dosimetry has the great advantage that the detector is very small and may therefore give good spatial resolution, especially if the detector is in the form of a teflon rod or disc. A further field of application is in situations where dose rate is very high and ion chambers cannot be used owing to recombination.

An interesting application of thermoluminescent dosimetry is in the dating of pottery samples in archaeological work. The pottery usually contains small grains of quartz which exhibit thermoluminescence. Firing of the pottery in manufacture resets the thermoluminescent clock in the quartz; after firing, natural radioactivity in the pottery itself and the soil in which it is buried causes the quartz to accumulate a dose which can be determined by heating a small sample.

Photographic dosimetry

A photographic emulsion consists of a suspension of small silver halide crystals in gelatin. The silver halide is usually silver bromide but it may have small amounts of additive, such as silver iodide, to influence the sensitivity of the emulsion. The size of the silver bromide crystals varies from about 0.3 μm to about 3 μm depending on the intended use of the emulsion. The emulsion is coated as a thin layer, usually on both sides of a plastic base or, for nuclear research, on one side of a glass plate. The emulsion layer is often covered with a thin coating of gelatin to protect it from abrasion.

During irradiation of the emulsion with ionizing radiation free electrons and holes are produced in the silver bromide lattice in a similar fashion to the production of electrons and holes in a thermoluminescent material. When the electrons are trapped at lattice sites electrostatic forces cause Ag^+ ions from the lattice to migrate to the trapped electrons, neutralizing their charge and causing the deposition of small amounts of metallic silver at the trapping sites. It is these small agglomerations of silver atoms which are the latent image. In the process of development solutions of organic reducing agents are used to convert Ag^+ ions in the crystal to metallic silver, the reaction occurring more rapidly in the crystals that form the latent image. By suitable choice of developing conditions it is possible to attain a high degree of discrimination between the crystals of the latent image and those that have not absorbed radiation. The degree of development, and hence the amount of silver deposited, is influenced not only by the composition of the developer but also by the time and temperature of development and for this reason development is usually standardized. Subsequent to development undeveloped crystals are dissolved with a fixing solution of sodium thiosulphate to render the image permanent.

The blackening of the developed image is measured by its density. Density is defined by the attenuation of a beam of white light in the image. If the intensity of the beam is I_0 in the absence of the film and I when the film is introduced into the beam, then the density is defined by

$$D = \log_{10}(I_0/I)$$

Density is an additive quantity. If a double coated film has a density D_1 in one emulsion layer and D_2 in the other the total density is $D_1 + D_2$. Even an area of the emulsion which has received no radiation will show a certain density called the background or fog density. The net density of an area of the emulsion is the total density minus the fog density; it is the density produced by exposure to the radiation.

The photographic emulsion is not an absolute dosemeter and must be calibrated against some other system such as an ionization chamber.

If the net density produced in an emulsion by X-rays is measured for different exposures (measured in roentgens) it is found that the density increases with exposure as shown in fig. 55. At very high exposures the density may pass through a maximum and then decrease with increasing exposure, an effect known as solarization. This implies that at high exposures a photographic emulsion cannot be used to determine exposure unambiguously since a particular density may correspond to two different

Fig. 55

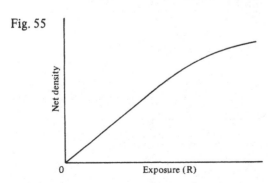

exposures. With low exposures the net density is proportional to the exposure, but the extent of the proportional region depends on the radiation used and the nature of the emulsion.

The sensitivity of an emulsion is defined as the reciprocal of either the exposure or dose needed to produce a given net density in the emulsion. In this context dose may be a more difficult quantity to determine since the inhomogeneity of the emulsion leads to a different dose to the silver bromide crystals and the gelatin matrix. The density chosen for the measurement of sensitivity depends on the application of the emulsion. In diagnostic radiology the net density is usually chosen as 1.0 since this represents a reasonable average of the densities produced in a typical radiograph. In the use of film for personnel monitoring the net density may be chosen as 0.3 since this is a better measure of typical levels produced in such films. Sensitivity is frequently used in a relative sense to compare the response of two films to the same radiation or the same film to different radiations.

The sensitivity of an emulsion depends on a number of factors; apart from the purely photographic factors such as emulsion type and development conditions it depends on the LET of the radiation and may depend to some extent on the angle of incidence of the radiation on the emulsion. With photons the relative sensitivity varies by a large factor, depending on the effective energy of the photons (fig. 56), since the photons must first interact with the emulsion to produce secondary electrons and it is these secondary electrons which produce the latent image. With photons above about 200 keV most of the interaction is by the Compton process and the sensitivity of the emulsion does not vary much with energy, but at lower energies the photoelectric process is the predominant interaction because the atomic numbers of silver

Fig. 56

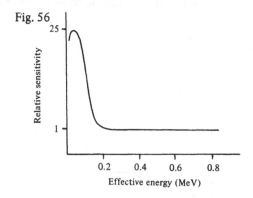

and bromine are relatively high (47 and 35 respectively) and consequently there is a marked increase in the sensitivity of the emulsion. At low energies the sensitivity of the emulsion may be of the order of twenty to thirty times higher than at high energies. This marked variation of sensitivity with energy makes it difficult to use emulsions for precise measurement of exposure or dose when working with photons. The main field of application of photographic emulsions is in personnel monitoring where high precision may not be required.

Films used for personnel monitoring should be capable of measuring in two distinct situations. They should be able to record the low levels of radiation that are received under normal working conditions and also the levels received in the few accidentally high exposures which, even with the best will in the world, do seem to happen occasionally. These two types of exposure require different characteristics of the film. To measure small exposures the film needs to have high sensitivity to produce a measurable density, but if a film of this type is given a high exposure the density is so high that it is difficult to determine the exposure with any degree of precision, so, for the few accidental high exposures, the film needs to have a low sensitivity. To meet both requirements the film may be manufactured with emulsions having different characteristics on its two surfaces, the sensitivity of one being about ten times that of the other. 'Normal' exposures produce most of the blackening in the sensitive emulsion. To measure accidentally high exposures the high sensitivity emulsion is stripped off after development and the low sensitivity emulsion is used to determine the exposure.

For measurement of exposure to photons the variation of sensitivity of the emulsion with photon energy poses a problem. In a fortnight (the period for which a monitoring film is commonly worn) the person who has worn the film may have been exposed to photons with a range of energies. In a typical hospital the wearer may have been exposed to photons from an X-ray set in a diagnostic radiology department working at, say, 80 kVp and to X-rays from a set working at 200 kVp in a therapy department and also to ^{60}Co gamma rays. The film has a different sensitivity to each of these radiations, but it is necessary to estimate the total dose received in the fortnight. There are three possible approaches to this problem. The film can be used in conjunction with a scintillator, so that the photons interact with the scintillator producing light and the blackening of the film is produced predominantly by this light. In this system the primary interaction of the photons is with the scintillator, which may be more nearly air equivalent than the film and show little variation of light output with exposure at different photon energies. The disadvantages of this system are that it may show a variation of sensitivity with angle of incidence of the radiation (due to the variation of effective thickness of the scintillator at different angles of incidence) and that the amount of blackening may depend not only on the total amount of light but also on the time the film is exposed to it, an effect known as reciprocity failure. An alternative approach is to sandwich the film between two filters of, say, tin. The object of the tin filters is to attenuate low energy photons by the photoelectric process to a greater extent than the high energy photons, thus compensating for the enhanced sensitivity of the emulsion to low energy photons. The limitation of this technique is that the differential attenuation in the filter for high and low energy photons depends on the angle of incidence of the radiation, since the thickness of filter traversed by the radiation varies with its angle of incidence.

In both of these methods the objective is to alter the response of the film so that the combination of film and scintillator or film and filter gives a flatter response to photons of different energy. A better approach is to accept the variation of film sensitivity with photon energy as it stands but to adopt a procedure which allows the energy of the photons to be determined, so that

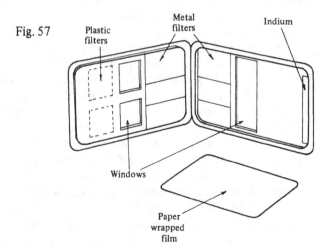

Fig. 57   Plastic filters   Metal filters   Indium

Windows

Paper wrapped film

the correct sensitivity can be used to estimate the exposure. To
this end, the film, which is contained in a light-tight paper envelope, is sandwiched between an array of filters of different thicknesses and materials in a plastic holder (fig. 57). The centre of the
film is situated between windows in the plastic holder so that
radiation may reach the film in this area without any filtration at
all. One end of the holder has thin plastic filters of the same
material as the holder and the other end of the holder contains
filters of, for example, tin and aluminium of different thicknesses.
After development the density of the film can be measured under
the window and the different filters. From the differences of
density it is possible to deduce the type of radiation and estimate
its energy so that the correct sensitivity of the film can be used to
determine the dose received by the wearer. For the measurement
of neutrons the film holder contains a strip of cadmium or
indium and the blackening produced under this strip by the products of neutron induced reactions in it is used to measure the
dose of neutrons.

8. Radiation protection

Most of the effects of ionizing radiations on biological systems are harmful to them. This unembroidered statement needs some elaboration since there are a number of instances, particularly in medicine, where the use of these radiations is obviously beneficial. There are two main medical applications of ionizing radiations: in radiotherapy and diagnosis.

Radiotherapy is the treatment of malignant disease by ionizing radiation. The objective of the treatment is to destroy malignant cells without, so far as is possible, producing harmful effects in healthy tissues. The overall effect of a successful therapeutic treatment is the survival of the patient, but, nevertheless, the direct effects of the radiation have been harmful in that the cells have been destroyed. The ideal condition of causing no harm to healthy tissues cannot be realized in practice because healthy tissue is invariably irradiated to a certain extent together with the malignant cells and so a certain amount of damage is also produced in it. Although the overall effect on the patient is clearly beneficial, at the cellular level the effects of the radiation are detrimental.

The use of ionizing radiations in diagnosis is to investigate conditions within the patient either by the differential attenuation of X-rays from an external source or by the distribution of a suitable radioactive material when introduced into the body. Though the radiation may produce some harmful effects in the patient, the overall effect is beneficial since the use of the radiation allows the diagnosis of conditions which would otherwise be left untreated.

These two types of medical irradiation are fairly clear-cut in that the beneficial effects to the patient outweigh any harmful effects, but looked at from a broader viewpoint the situation may not be so unequivocal. In irradiating patients in radiotherapy or diagnosis not only the patient is irradiated but also the personnel administering the radiation and, to a lesser extent, the general public, and due consideration must be given to the levels of radiation they receive. Personnel are irradiated since, if they are administering an external beam of X-rays or γ-rays and are controlling the irradiation from a separate room, some of the radiation which is scattered from the patient and the structure of the room in which the patient is situated will, to a certain extent, penetrate the walls of the room in which the operator is working, owing to the exponential nature of the attenuation of the radiation. Similarly members of the general public are irradiated as they walk past the treatment room in the corridors of the hospital or in roads outside the building. In administering radioactive isotopes both the administrator and the general public are irradiated. In this case the main hazard to the general public is in the disposal of the radioactive material, either as surplus solution or as radioactive excreta from the patient. This waste material may be disposed of in the main sewage system and, after treatment in the sewage-works, the effluent is released into a river or the sea whence, depending on its half-life, some of the radioactive content may find its way into the populace as food or water.

Whenever ionizing radiations are used, either as beams of radiation produced by accelerating particles or as the emissions from radioactive materials, whether they are used in hospitals, in research, in industry or for educational purposes, they present a danger to the user and to the general public and, in hospitals, to the patient. The field of measurement and control of these hazards is known as radiation protection. The field of radiation protection is vast and the subject can only be touched upon in a book of this scope. The reader is strongly recommended to consult the publications listed in the bibliography.

The biological effects of ionizing radiations

The biological effects of radiations may be classified in various ways. For instance they may be divided into stochastic effects, the probability of which occurring is a function of the dose, and non-stochastic effects, the severity of which varies with the dose. In dealing with radiation protection it is convenient to group them in two classes: somatic effects and genetic effects. Somatic effects are effects which are produced in the body tissues, that is, tissues which have developed to perform specialized functions. Genetic effects are effects produced by the radiation in germ cells, the reproductive cells which, at a later date, may combine and differentiate to produce adult individuals.

Examples of the harmful somatic effects of radiation are the depression of the red blood cell count, the production of eye cataracts (a non-stochastic effect) and the induction of a number of malignant conditions such as leukaemia (a stochastic effect). The severity of many somatic effects, rather than the probability of their occurrence, may depend on the dose of radiation received, the duration of the irradiation, whether the dose is delivered as a number of fractions spread over a period of time, and the total volume of tissue irradiated. As an example, if the hand is given a single short duration dose of 5 Gy the skin will react soon after the irradiation and turn red, but if the same dose is given in separate fractions spread over a long period there may be no obvious effect. If, alternatively, the whole body is irradiated with a dose of 5 Gy there is a high probability that death will shortly ensue. Effects like these often show a threshold dose level below which they do not occur. Induction of malignancies is thought to behave rather differently, the probability of their occurrence being proportional to the total dose received.

The genetic effects of ionizing radiation are due to mutations in genes and other chromosomal changes of the germ cells. The main difference between genetic effects and somatic effects is that, apart from social consequences, somatic effects affect only the irradiated individual whereas genetic effects do not affect this person but may appear in future generations, possibly many generations after the irradiation. At the dose levels met with in radiation protection genetic effects are regarded as stochastic effects and are treated as though their incidence is proportional to dose.

It may be argued that genetic effects are not necessarily harmful and may in fact be beneficial since new and 'better' types of the species may be produced. This is unlikely to be the case since mutations occur spontaneously and natural selection has tended to weed out those mutants which are poorly adapted to survive. Although the spontaneous mutation rate is not high, during the many generations that man has existed the species has tended to become better adapted to its environment and radiation induced mutations are therefore likely to be deleterious.

The ethics of radiation protection

The underlying ethic of radiation protection is that everyone using ionizing radiation has a moral obligation both to themselves and the rest of the population, both present and future, to ensure their safety from the effects of radiation. In many advanced countries this obligation is reinforced by legislation.

It might seem that the only way of preventing the harmful effects of radiations is to ban their use entirely, but this extreme measure would be rather illogical since every member of the population is irradiated to a certain extent by cosmic radiation and by radiation from naturally occurring radioactive materials in the earth's crust and in their own bodies. In practice a more reasonable approach is adopted and the hazards of radiation are treated in the same way as all the other hazards of life, the risks from the

radiation being balanced against the benefits that accrue from
their use. With this approach the principles of radiation protection
are that ionizing radiations are not used unless there is a net
benefit from their use. They are not used when the effect can be
achieved more safely by some other means, and when they are
used the dose received by personnel using them and members of
the general population is limited to a sufficiently low value that
effects which show a threshold with dose are not produced and
effects such as carcinogenesis and the genetic effect, the probability of which occurring is proportional to the total dose
received, are reduced to an acceptable level.

Dose limitation

In order to specify a limiting dose that may be applied universally
to the various types of ionizing radiation that are used, some
means must be found to specify an equivalent dose of the different
radiations. This is necessary since the biological effects of radiations
depend not only on the dose but also on the microscopic distribution of energy in the irradiated tissue and therefore on the LET
of the radiation. Thus the biological effect of a given dose of radiation varies with its LET.

The dose-equivalent (H) for a particular type of irradiation is
defined by

$$H = DQN$$

where D is the dose in grays, Q is the quality factor, which depends
on the LET of the radiation, and N is a factor depending on other
modifying influences such as dose rate and fractionation of the
dose. At present N is assigned the value unity. The quality factor
Q is illustrated in fig. 58. The effectiveness of other radiations is
compared with that of low LET radiations such as X-rays. From
this curve we see that fast neutrons are about ten times as effective
in producing a biological effect as X-rays and alpha particles about
twenty times as effective.

Since N is taken as unity, we have the dose-equivalent equal to
the product of the dose in grays and the quality factor. Dose-
equivalent has a special unit called the sievert (Sv). Since the quality factor is a plain number the units of the sievert are the same as
the gray, i.e. joules per kilogram. In older literature another unit
will be found called the rem, which is similar to the sievert but is
based on the older unit of dose, the rad. Since 1 Gy equals 100
rads, 1 Sv equals 100 rems.

With this definition of dose-equivalent for different types of radiation a limit can be set to the amount of radiation that can be received in order that the biological effects induced by the radiation in the body will be at an acceptable level. The recommended dose-equivalent limit for workers exposed occupationally to radiation from external sources is 50 mSv per year, corresponding to 1 mSv per week or a constant dose-equivalent rate of 25 μSv per hour, assuming a 50 week working year and a 40 hour working week and that the dose rate is constant throughout the working period.

When radioactive isotopes enter the body, either accidentally by ingestion or inhalation, or deliberately in medical procedures, the situation is more complicated than irradiation from external sources. The complications arise from three factors. The first is a biological factor, depending on the metabolism of the isotope in the body. Metabolism may cause the isotope to be concentrated in certain organs or tissues, in which case these organs or tissues will be more heavily irradiated than if the isotope were distributed uniformly throughout the body. An example of metabolic concentration occurs when isotopes of strontium or radium enter the body. Since their chemical nature is similar to that of calcium they tend to be concentrated in the bone of the subject. Metabolism will also cause the isotope to be excreted; the more rapid the excretion the less time it spends in the body and consequently the smaller the dose it delivers. The other two factors are physical, depending on the half-life of the isotope and the nature of its emissions. The half-life of the isotope affects the hazard since, for a given activity, the number of radioative nuclei present is directly proportional to the half-life and so a given activity of a long-lived

Fig. 58

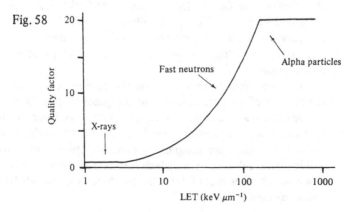

isotope presents a greater hazard than the same activity of an isotope with a short half-life. The nature of the emissions also
influences the hazard since the distribution of dose is dependent
on both the energy of the radiation and the way in which it is
absorbed in matter. In this respect alpha particles emitted inside
the body present a very serious hazard, especially if the isotope
producing them is concentrated in a specific region, because the
range of the particles is very short and all their energy is deposited
close to the site where they are produced, leading to a high local
dose. The net hazard from radioactive isotopes within the body
is due to a combination of these three factors, the metabolism of
the isotope, its half-life and the nature of its emissions. Protection
from internal exposure from radioactive material is based on
annual limits of intake (ALI) which vary from isotope to isotope.

Protective measures from external irradiation
Irradiation of the body by an external beam of radiation may
arise from the use of a particle accelerator, such as an X-ray set,
or from the use of a high activity radioactive source, such as a
cobalt-60 unit, to produce a beam of γ-rays, or in the manipulation of relatively low activity radioactive sources during experimental or clinical procedures. The dose-equivalent due to external
irradiation can be limited in two ways. Since dose is the product
of dose rate and time, the dose-equivalent can be limited by
controlling either the dose rate or the time of exposure to the
radiation.

Limitation of the dose rate can be achieved in two ways, either
by increasing the distance from the source or by attenuating the
radiation by interposing suitable protective barriers between the
source of radiation and people working in its vicinity. Frequently
a combination of both measures is used simultaneously. An
example of the use of distance alone is in the handling of weak
radioactive sources. The sources are not touched with the hands
since this would cause a high dose rate at the fingers where they
contact the source, owing to the inverse square law variation of
dose rate. Instead the source is manipulated with long forceps to
keep the source as far away from the body as practicable, thus
reducing the dose rate. The limit to the length of forceps that can
be used is about a metre and in handling strong sources this distance would not reduce the dose rate sufficiently to afford
adequate protection, and so a combination of distance and a protective barrier is used. The source is manipulated behind a barrier

of either lead or steel and remotely controlled tongs are used for the manipulation.

The material used for a protective barrier depends on the nature of the radiation being protected against and the dose rate. Alpha particles from a radioactive source can be protected against quite easily since their range in air is of the order of only a few centimetres and, provided the source is kept at a greater distance from the body, none of the particles can reach it. Beta particles present a greater danger since their ranges may be of the order of metres of air, but, since they have a finite range in matter, they can be protected against by a barrier of the order of a few centimetres thick of a low atomic number material such as perspex. Gamma rays from a radioactive source or X-rays from a particle accelerator present a much more difficult protection problem because they do not have a finite range but are attenuated exponentially. With this type of radiation the thickness of the barrier and material from which it is constructed should be such that the dose rate outside the barrier is reduced to an acceptable level. In designing such barriers the aim should be to reduce the dose-equivalent rate to less than 25 μSv per hour. A certain amount of flexibility is allowed in the choice of level of dose rate outside the barrier since the limit of dose-equivalent is specified on an annual basis at 50 mSv per year and hence if the dose-equivalent rate is more than 25 μSv per hour it is acceptable to use the time of occupation of the site to control the dose-equivalent. Occupancy factors may be used in hospitals where the setting-up time for a patient in either X-ray therapy or diagnosis may be an appreciable fraction of the total time of the treatment. Occupancy factors must be used with prudence since it is often not possible to control the time of occupation.

The material used for protective barriers depends largely on the photon energy and may also depend on economic factors. The cheapest way of providing adequate protection is to use conventional building materials and have the barriers erected as part of the fabric of the building during its construction. Any further modification of the barriers is likely to be an expensive exercise. In the low energy region of X-ray diagnosis normal building materials such as bricks and mortar may suffice, provided that modern light-weight aggregate blocks are not used. If the attenuation of a normal wall is insufficient it can be increased by coating it with a layer of high atomic number material, using the high photoelectric attenuation in the low energy region ($\tau \propto Z^4$) to reduce the dose rate. These coatings may be of barium plaster (in which the calcium content of normal plaster is replaced with higher atomic number barium) or of lead. Protection in the diagnostic energy region can be achieved relatively easily and provided the radiographer is not in the primary X-ray beam and stands behind a screen of lead about 1 mm thick she can safely be in the treatment room during the exposure.

Adequate protection in the therapy energy range is more difficult to provide, partly because the exposure times are much longer and partly because the radiation is more penetrating. In this energy range attenuation of both the primary beam and scattered radiation is mainly by the Compton process and therefore using high atomic number materials has no great advantage. Protection is most cheaply provided by using normal concrete, the aim being to impose an adequate mass per unit area of attenuating material between the source and surrounding work areas. If concrete is used for the construction of the protective barriers it must be sufficiently compacted by vibration during the casting process to prevent the formation of voids. The minimum thickness of a barrier depends on the intensity of the radiation incident upon it and the penetrating power of the radiation. In general, the primary beam of radiation is of much greater intensity and penetrating power than radiation scattered from the patient or structure of the room. Consequently barriers which are irradiated by the primary photon beam must be considerably thicker than barriers which can receive only scattered radiation. The lower penetrating power of scattered radiation is due to the photons scattered in the Compton process having lower energy than the incident photons. Since it is often difficult to construct doors which afford a high degree of protection they are normally sited in the treatment room at a point where they can receive only scattered radiation. In order to prevent accidental entry into the treatment room while the source is switched on the door is interlocked in such a way that either the door cannot be opened while the source is on or, alternatively, opening the door a very small amount automatically switches the source off. In the therapy range there is no possibility of the source of radiation being controlled from within the treatment room and the control desk is situated in a separate cubicle outside the treatment room in a position to where the primary beam of radiation cannot be directed. In order to view the patient a window is built into the wall between the control cubicle and the treatment room. Depending on the nature of the radiation source, this window may be constructed of thick lead glass (glass which has lead salts added to increase its power of absorption) or may be a periscopic device. With high energy, high dose rate machines, viewing may be accomplished by closed circuit television, thus minimizing the size of apertures in the barriers.

Protective measures from internal irradiation

Internal irradiation arises from radioactive isotopes introduced into the body either deliberately in medical procedures or accidentally in the manipulation of unsealed sources.

In medical procedures protection of the patient is accomplished by a suitable choice of isotope and, if the isotope is used for diagnostic purposes, the sensitivity of the detecting system. The choice is made by selecting an isotope and detector sensitivity which enables the minimum dose to be delivered to the patient consistent with being able to produce the desired effect or acquiring the desired information.

Protection from accidentally ingested or inhaled radioactive material can only be achieved by reducing the risk of ingestion or inhalation. To this end rubber or plastic gloves are always worn when handling active materials and, if necessary, non-absorbent protective clothing. During manipulation care is taken not to touch the rest of the body with the hands, particularly around the face. At the end of the procedure the gloves are removed and the hands monitored with a Geiger counter or scintillation counter to check their freedom from activity and, if necessary, are thoroughly washed and remonitored. Containers of active solutions are manipulated in large trays which are capable of containing the whole solution in case of accidental spillage and these trays are lined with plastic-backed absorbent material.

If the processes carried out with the solution are capable of liberating active material into the atmosphere, or if the active material is in the form of a powder, the processing is carried out in a forced-draught fume cupboard. A cardinal rule of hygiene when using unsealed radioactive materials is that one does not eat, drink or smoke in laboratories where these materials are handled.

In order to protect the population at large from ingested radioactive material, the activities that may be disposed of in the drains are strictly controlled and it may be necessary to store material for a suitable time to allow it to decay before disposal. Long-lived isotopes which present a serious hazard to the population owing to the nature of their emissions or their metabolism are normally delivered to a competent authority for disposal.

Monitoring

Unlike many of the hazards of everyday life the dangers of ionizing radiations are insidious since the radiations cannot normally be sensed by the human body. The only method of ensuring safety from their effects is by measurement of the amounts of radiation, combined with intelligent working procedures. Measurement falls into two classes: departmental monitoring and personnel monitoring.

The objective of departmental monitoring is to ensure that the dose rate in the environs of radiation sources is sufficiently low that nobody is likely to exceed the limit of dose-equivalent. Measurements are usually made using portable high sensitivity ionization chambers. These chambers are of relatively large volume, of the order of a litre, since the limiting dose-equivalent rate is fairly low. Measurements must always be made on new installations and should be given top priority on completion of the installation. Such measurements are essential since the factors involved in the design of protective barriers are often not known very precisely and the designer may have to resort to experience and intuition.

Radiation surveys should be carried out under the worse possible conditions, for example if a number of radiation sources can be used simultaneously the radiation levels should be measured with all the sources in operation. If the protective barriers are found to be inadequate their absorptive power may have to be augmented or alternatively the direction in which the beam of radiation may point may have to be mechanically restricted. The scope of the survey should include not only rooms on the same floor as the radiation source but also those on floors above and below it. A radiation survey should also be carried out when old apparatus is replaced with new equipment in existing treatment rooms or if the procedure of irradiation is changed significantly.

In a radiation survey the dose rate at places where people work is measured. Personnel monitoring measures the dose they actually receive. In many countries it is obligatory for personnel who are likely to be exposed to more than thirty per cent of the annual dose-equivalent limit to wear a radiation dosemeter. A record must be kept of the doses received throughout the working life. The

radiation dosemeter may take various forms; the pocket ionization chamber described on p. 78 may be used or, more commonly, the film badge described on p. 100. The advantage of
using the ionization chamber is that it gives a reading at any time
whereas the film badge has to be processed before measurement.
The disadvantage of the ion chamber is that it has a limited range,
usually of the order of the maximum dose people are likely to
receive in a week, and cannot be used outside this range. Furthermore it is subject to accidental discharge which may be caused by
small bits of fluff or dust inside it. Consequently if the reading is
more than full scale one is never certain if this is due to radiation
or not.

The advantage of the film method of monitoring is that, provided the processing is carried out correctly there is usually little
doubt that the density of the film is due to radiation. A serious
limitation of the film badge method is that its sensitivity varies
markedly with the energy of the radiation and this sometimes
makes it difficult to make precise measurements; often it is not
possible to make measurements with an accuracy as high as ten
per cent.

A modern replacement of the film badge monitor is the use of
lithium fluoride thermoluminescent dosemeters. A lithium
fluoride monitor has a number of advantages compared with the
photographic monitor. Its sensitivity is fairly constant over a wide
range of radiation energies since the effective atomic number of
the dosemeter is fairly close to that of tissue, and the accuracy of
measurements is of the order of three per cent. It can be used to
measure a wide range of doses without the necessity for any
special processing. It is re-usable and the read-out process can be
automated thus reducing labour costs and, further, the signal from
the reader can be fed to a computer to store information on the
dose measured.

Bibliography

F.H. Attix, W.C. Roesch and E. Tochilin, *Radiation Dosimetry*, vols. 1 and 2. Academic Press, New York and London, 1968.

H.E. Johns and J.R. Cunningham, *The Physics of Radiology*. C.C. Thomas, Springfield, Illinois, 1969.

Code of Practice for the Protection of Persons against Ionizing Radiations arising from Medical and Dental Use. HMSO, London, 1972.

Guidance Notes for the Protection of Persons Exposed to Ionising Radiations in Research and Teaching. HMSO, London, 1976.

Recommendations of the International Commission on Radiological Protection, ICRP Publication 26. Pergamon Press, Oxford, 1977.

Index